An

Introduction

to

Quality

Improvement

in

Health

Care

Joint Commission Mission

The mission of the Joint Commission on Accreditation of Healthcare Organizations is to improve the quality of health care provided to the public. The Joint Commission develops standards of quality in collaboration with health professionals and others and stimulates health care organizations to meet or exceed the standards through accreditation and the teaching of quality improvement concepts.

Requests for permission to make copies of any part of this work should be mailed to: Permissions Editor, Department of Publications, Joint Commission on Accreditation of Healthcare Organizations, One Renaissance Boulevard, Oakbrook Terrace, IL 60181.

Address orders to: Customer Service Center, Joint Commisssion on Accreditation of Healthcare Organizations, One Renaissance Boulevard, Oakbrook Terrace, IL 60181.

Address editorial correspondence: Department of Publications, Joint Commission on Accreditation of Healthcare Organizations, One Renaissance Boulevard, Oakbrook Terrace, IL 60181.

CONTENTS

PREFACE

The approach to improving quality in health care is changing, motivated by both external and internal forces. Externally, payors, government, and the public are demanding accountability for the cost and quality of care. Internally, health care practitioners and administrators, as always, strive to improve quality and resources. In addition, health care organizations desire to make quality improvement something *they* initiate and conduct rather than something done to please external groups.

A greater understanding of quality improvement has accompanied these motivating forces. Quality-improvement theories and techniques—with special attention to the efforts of American Industry to make use of the quality-improvement processes that have revolutionized Japanese industry—are the subject of a growing body of research and writing. And the Joint Commission continues its Agenda for Change initiatives, which are designed to make future accreditation an effective stimulus for continuous improvement in the performance of health care organizations.

The upshot of this effort and knowledge is a move toward *quality improvement*. This approach

> ...acknowledges the humanity and complexity of health care organizations. Although individual competence and performance remain important, good patient care and acceptable (or better) outcomes are viewed as the product of all individual actions *and interactions* that relate directly or indirectly to the care received by the patient. Performance is thus a reflection of a variety of internal organization systems and subsystems that underlie essential day-to-day functions. Human error may occur within these often complex systems, but remedial actions are usually most appropriately directed to the system, not the human.[1]

Although identifying and solving isolated problems will always be a concern, quality improvement recognizes that the more significant advances will result from focusing on important functions and processes in order to improve the norm of performance.

The Joint Commission is taking direct action to assist health care organizations in implementing quality improvement. The Accreditation Manual for Hospitals is being reorganized around important functions rather than on isolated department and service structure. New standards are being developed to describe effective leadership and quality-improvement techniques. Clinical indicators are being developed and tested to use in quality assessment and improvement. And educational programs and publications, such as this one, are illuminating the transition from quality assurance to quality improvement.

An Introduction to Quality Improvement in Health Care is designed to facilitate the transition. It covers

- the evolution of approaches to quality that have given rise to quality improvement;
- the principles of quality improvement;
- the application of quality improvement to health care;
- methods to put quality improvement into action; and
- techniques of monitoring, assessing, and improving the quality of health care.

Another important focus of this book is the Joint Commission's revised quality standards. The revisions are explained in detail, and three appendixes present new standards and some ideas on the direction future standards are likely to take.

Quality improvement offers respect for the practitioner, understanding of the scope of activities that affect quality, and solid tools to assess and improve care. Fully implementing quality improvement is an extended process. It requires leadership commitment and resources such as time and expertise. The experience of organizations who have begun the implementation suggests that these efforts also have accompanying satisfactions: the pleasure of taking constructive action, improvement in performance, and savings of time and money.[2] Quality improvement is just beginning to be attempted by health care organizations. This book offers a formative report. As revised Joint Commission standards are in place and organizations gain experience with quality improvement, subsequent reports will provide an updated perspective on the challenges and successes of quality improvement in health care.

REFERENCES

1. O'Leary DS: CQI—A step beyond QA. Joint Commission Perspectives, Mar/Apr 1990.

2. Berwick DM: Curing Health Care, New Strategies for Quality Improvement. San Francisco: Jossey-Bass Publishers, 1990.

CHAPTER ONE

WHY A TRANSITION TO QUALITY IMPROVEMENT?

The health care system is engaged in a high-stakes search for a better solution to its quality dilemma.... Growing naturally out of the steady progression from implicit peer review to medical audits to systematic quality assurance..., the philosophies and methods of formalized continuous quality improvement...are thought by many to answer this need.[1]

The body of literature on quality improvement is growing; health care organizations are beginning to implement quality improvement, based in part on lessons learned from Japanese industry; revised Joint Commission standards will embrace the concept of quality improvement. Clearly, a transition is under way, but the question still must be asked: why move from quality assurance to quality improvement?

The pressure on health care organizations today to reduce or control costs and to maintain and demonstrate quality has provided strong incentive to improve the means by which quality is assessed and improved. Perceived difficulties with current systems and innovative techniques observed in Japanese industry have provided direction to the efforts. Quality improvement, a central pillar of the Joint Commission's Agenda for Change, is the result.

Viewed out of context, such a transition could seem abrupt—a "conversion to a new religion" or adoption of "the latest fad—"but when viewed within the progression of health care quality assessment techniques in the last four decades, quality improvement is clearly a natural outgrowth of arduous study and experience.[1] The transition from quality assurance to quality improvement is an inevitable step in the evolution of approaches to managing health care quality. Figure 1 (page 8) illustrates the evolution of the Joint Commission's quality standards and the health care field's approaches to assessing and improving quality.

THE EVOLUTION

Those who have followed Joint Commission standards—particularly the quality assurance standards—for the past decades will have noticed the evolution in approaches toward defining, measuring, and improving the quality of health care. From 1953 (the year the first Joint Commission standards were published) through the early 1970s, the standards referred in general terms to assessing and improving the quality of care, but did not suggest specific methodologies for the activities. Hospitals did carry out reviews, especially morbidity and mortality review, that generally examined specific cases for questionable practice.

Audits

In 1975 the Quality of Professional Services standard was published, requiring hospitals to "demonstrate that the quality of patient care was consistently optimal by continually evaluating care through reliable and valid measures."[2] The assumptions implicit in this statement are important and would remain for some time in quality-related writing and activity. The word "optimal" suggests it is possible to improve the quality of care to the point that it is the best that possibly can be expected under the circumstances. In other words, the implication is that an end level of improvement exists, an ideal level of quality. The term "consistently" makes it clear that this ideal level of care should be achieved at all times

EVOLUTION OF APPROACHES
TO QUALITY ASSESSMENT

IMPLICIT REVIEW
(Morbidity and Mortality Review)

TIME LIMITED STUDIES
(Retrospective Audits)

ONGOING MONITORING AND EVALUATION
(Quality Assurance)

INTEGRATED PROGRAM OF CONTINUAL IMPROVEMENT
(Quality Improvement/Agenda for Change)

Figure 1

How the approaches to assessing and improving health care, and the relevant Joint Commission standards, have evolved.

throughout the organization. "Demonstrate" suggests that this optimal care can be documented, and that this documentation could be shown to the appropriate parties on request. "Continually" indicates that efforts to achieve this level of quality would be ongoing. And "reliable and valid measures" asks, for the first time, that objective methods be established to examine and document quality.

The standard went on to require explicit, measurable criteria. These criteria were to be used in retrospective, outcome-focused, time-limited audits of care. Unfortunately, the data were seldom put to use in systematic efforts to improve care. The data themselves were not helpful without a systematic process for identifying areas to assess, evaluating the data, and taking actions to improve care.

In response to shortcomings of the audit procedure, the Joint Commission in 1979 approved a quality assurance chapter to replace the Quality of Professional Service standard. Unlike the previous standards, the quality assurance standards emphasized the value of a coordinated, organizationwide quality assurance program. They also allowed hospitals greater flexibility in the methods they could choose to assess and improve the quality of care. In addition, the

standards emphasized focusing quality assurance activities on problems whose solution would have a significant effect on patient care outcomes.

The move toward a systematic, organizationwide effort to improve quality was a significant step, and the problem-focused approach was amenable to morbidity and mortality review and other established review activities in hospitals. Many hospitals, however, had difficulty designing and implementing effective methods to assess and improve the quality of care.

Ongoing Monitoring and Evaluation

Revision to the quality assurance standards in 1985 continued to emphasize the organizationwide quality assurance program, but replaced the problem-focused approach with systematic monitoring and evaluation of important aspects of patient care. It was believed that a more comprehensive, ongoing program of monitoring would "plug the holes" that a strictly problem-focused approach would leave. By choosing their important aspects of care, continually collecting data on performance, and taking necessary actions to solve problems or otherwise improve care, hospitals could reasonably expect to "assure" quality.

The standards asked that the systematic monitoring and evaluation be performed in specific hospital departments or services, including nursing, anesthesia, radiology, emergency, and others. The standards also included a number of tailored quality assurance activities, to be performed primarily by the medical staff: medical staff departmental review, drug usage evaluation, surgical case review, blood usage review, medical record review, and the pharmacy and therapeutics function.

The health care field continued to request assistance with methodology. Exactly how should important aspects of care be selected? What kind of data should be collected and by whom? How could quality and appropriateness be objectively evaluated? What kind of actions should be taken? What kind of documentation was necessary?

The ten-step process. Faced with these important questions, the Joint Commission began to formulate a detailed monitoring and evaluation process, whose by-now-familiar ten steps included assigning responsibility, identifying important aspects of care, identifying indicators to monitor the aspects of care, collecting data, evaluating care, and taking actions to improve care. The steps of this process soon became part of the quality assurance standards.

Difficulties. The health care field has been grappling for several years now with monitoring and evaluation and quality assurance, and that experience has been at once productive, frustrating, and enlightening. Quality proved an illusive concept, capable of being viewed from many perspectives; the notions of "assuring" quality and "optimal" care became less realistic as more was learned about quality. In addition, those carrying out quality assurance had difficulty knowing just what information could be collected to identify opportunities for improvement. The methods of assessing, measuring, and improving quality seemed too subjective.

Also, despite standards that required an organizationwide program, quality tended to be the purview of a discrete department that found itself with the unenviable task of persuading already busy staff to take on more tasks. Further resentment was caused by the perception that quality assurance was performed only to placate external bodies, particularly the Joint Commission.

Monitoring and evaluation activities tended to be isolated, the boundaries delineated by the hospital departments and services. Although Joint Commission quality assurance standards stressed cooperation between departments, those same standards described the activities department by department in 14 separate chapters.

Despite these struggles, the interest of third-party payors, competition in the health care field, and the professional desire for self-improvement kept quality in the spotlight.

QUALITY IMPROVEMENT

Outside the health care field, quality also was in the spotlight. American industry had declined, while the Japanese had gained the reputation as manufacturers of remarkably high-quality products, especially automobiles and audiovisual equipment. The principles on which Japanese industrial success was founded were now gaining wider currency in America. These principles, which were championed, ironically, by Americans W. Edwards Deming and Joseph M. Juran, stress understanding the complex processes of any industry, measuring performance using reliable statistical methods, and using the information to build quality into the processes (rather than focusing exclusively on inspection). In addition, the importance of leadership is stressed; leaders must demonstrate their commitment to quality improvement by investing time and money in the process, by removing barriers to communication and improvement, and by creating an organizational culture that places quality at the highest level of importance.

Ultimately, the Japanese success rests on the concept that quality was something to be continually improved through the study and refinement of processes; it was not an optimal level of performance one could attain by searching out "bad apples" and removing them from the barrel.

American companies have begun to understand and adopt the Japanese method of quality improvement (often called "continuous quality improvement" or "total quality management"). And those concerned with quality in health care also began to ask whether the Japanese model could be adapted to health care.

A number of sources said "yes." For example, the National Demonstration Project on Quality Improvement in Health Care, which began in 1987, paired industrial quality experts with groups from various health care organizations. Each team formulated an issue to address using quality improvement techniques. The results show a high rate of success for the projects, and indicate the tools and principles of quality improvement can successfully involve leaders and staff, improve care and services, and save money.[3]

The application of quality improvement to health care is discussed in detail in Chapters Three through Six.

The Agenda for Change

The Joint Commission, for its part, launched the Agenda for Change—multi-year initiatives designed to make future accreditation an effective stimulus for continuous improvement in the performance of health care organizations. The Agenda for Change was initiated in 1987 and encompasses

- a refocusing of Joint Commission standards;
- improvements in survey and decision-making processes; and
- creation of an interactive data system based on well-tested indicators of an organization's performance.

The refocusing of standards in part is designed to facilitate implementation of quality improvement. More specifically, the Joint Commission's standards will be modified to

- highlight those governance, clinical, managerial, and support functions that most affect the quality of care and services—and, therefore, patient outcomes—(that is, *important functions*);
- emphasize the effective application of the wide variety of quality improvement tools to the assessment and improvement of an organization's performance of these important functions;

- retain and improve those structural requirements that help an organization effectively perform the important functions; and
- streamline and shorten the standards by removing irrelevant requirements and eliminating unnecessary duplication.

Coupled with improved standards will be an enhanced survey and decision-making process. Modification as a result of the Agenda for Change will

- increase the accuracy and consistency of the Joint Commission's evaluation of an organization's performance of the *important functions* described in the standards;
- improve the relevance and practical utility of the education provided by surveyors during the on-site visit;
- improve the efficiency of the pre-survey, on-site, and post-survey processes and, to the extent feasible, individualize each to the organization being surveyed;
- allow the surveyor, prior to the end of the on-site visit, to provide the organization with a preliminary report of observations and the overall level of standards compliance;
- allow return of a final survey report to the organization in a timely fashion (45 to 60 days); and
- allow provision of a final written report that (1) is consistent with the preliminary on-site report, (2) clearly identifies the organization's strengths and weaknesses, and (3) is helpful to the organization in setting priorities for improvement.

The Agenda for Change shifts how organizations are assessed. Up to now, by focusing on the structures and processes of the health care organization, the Joint Commission has been measuring the *capability* of the organization to provide high-quality care and services. Of course, only if the necessary structures (for example, people and equipment) are in place, and the plans for what they do (that is, the processes) are well designed, can high-quality care result. But the right structures and good designs for processes do not guarantee good care or results.

With changes in the standards and survey process, and the development of an indicator monitoring system, the Joint Commission will now be focusing on answering the following questions about the performance of the health care organization:

- Are the right, well-designed processes actually being carried out?
- Do the processes conform with nationally accepted standards?

- Does the organization make necessary improvements in both the design of the processes and in how well they are carried out?
- What are the results of the processes—including patient outcomes—and how do these results compare with those achieved by others?

The answers to these questions will be used primarily to assess how well the organization provides care, rather than primarily whether it is capable of providing good care.

Quality Assessment and Improvement Standards

Revisions in Joint Commission standards dealing with quality assessment and improvement are a vital part of the Agenda for Change. These standard revisions seek to build on the strong basis quality assurance has provided, especially its emphasis on reliable data, ongoing monitoring, maintaining improvement over time, and organizationwide involvement. The revisions are designed to remove some of the negative connotations of quality assurance: that a single level of quality can be guaranteed, that the focus should be on individuals rather than on processes, and that the activities are carried out for the sake of external entities such as the Joint Commission.

In the 1992 Accreditation Manual for Hospitals, the former "Quality Assurance" chapter is renamed "Quality Assessment and Improvement." Significant changes follow:

- The chapter includes a preamble that discusses the transition from quality assurance to quality improvement and explains that the standards are based on the principles of quality improvement.
- The preamble that formerly described the ten-step monitoring and evaluation process is deleted.
- The standards pertaining to the monitoring and evaluation process have been clarified.
- Barriers to organizationwide quality assessment and improvement have been removed.
- New standards QA.1 through QA.1.6 have been added, which address the roles of hospital leaders in continuous quality improvement.
- The requirement to use monthly meetings of the clinical departments of the medical staff as the only acceptable mechanism to consider monitoring and evaluation findings has been deleted.
- The phrase "quality assessment and improvement" has been substituted for "quality assurance."
- The phrase "and appropriateness" has been eliminated

from "monitoring and evaluating the quality and appropriateness of care" because contemporary definitions of quality include appropriateness as one of quality's characteristics.

- Requirements for surgical case review, drug usage evaluation, and blood usage review have been clarified.

The 1994 quality assessment and improvement standards will more fully incorporate principles and techniques that foster continuous improvement in performance and quality. These standards will be divided into five sections:

- Leadership responsibility for quality improvement;
- Techniques of quality improvement;
- Education and training;
- Communication and collaboration; and
- Evaluation of effectiveness of quality improvement activities.

The new and future standards and their implications for health care organizations are discussed further in Chapter Four.

THE TRANSITION

Quality assurance provides a solid base on which quality improvement can be built. Improved knowledge of quality-improvement techniques and the need to demonstrate high quality provide the impetus to change. Quality improvement incorporates the strengths of quality assurance, while broadening its scope, refining its approach to assessing and improving care, and dispensing with the negative connotations sometimes associated with quality assurance.

The Joint Commission is aware of the discomfort that accompanies change, and the other barriers, including lack of funds and personnel. Many important questions have been and will be raised by this transition. Among the most pressing are these:

- What exactly is quality improvement?
- How is quality improvement implemented in a health care organization?
- What are the time and financial costs of this change?
- What will become of monitoring and evaluation?
- What are the new standards?

This book will answer these questions and provide hospitals and other health care organizations with the basis to begin implementing the transition.

Chapter Two will discuss the principles of quality improvement in more detail.

REFERENCES

1. Roberts JS; Schyve PS: From QA to QI: The views and role of the Joint Commission. The Quality Letter, May 1990.

2. Joint Commission on Accreditation of Hospitals: Supplement to the Accreditation Manual for Hospitals. Chicago: Joint Commission, 1975.

3. Berwick DM: Curing Health Care, New Strategies for Quality Improvement San Francisco: Jossey-Bass Publishers, 1990.

Chapter Two

WHAT IS QUALITY IMPROVEMENT?

...[Q]uality improvement guided by theory and systematic information can help complex systems of production to function at levels of quality, efficiency, productivity, and morale that usually cannot even be imagined in systems "improved" by misguided intuition and habitual forms of control.[1]

Because quality improvement is a multi-faceted concept, a comprehensive understanding of its principles and characteristics is necessary if its implementation is to be effective.

This chapter will begin by presenting thoughts on quality improvement from several of its leading writers and thinkers—W. Edwards Deming, Joseph M. Juran, and Philip Crosby. From these thoughts, a summary of the key points of quality improvement will be constructed. How quality improvement applies to health care organizations, and how these organizations can put quality improvement into action, will be covered in Chapters Three and Four.

THE EXPERTS

This section offers of survey of how W. Edwards Deming, Joseph M. Juran, and Philip B. Crosby articulate the principles and characteristics of quality improvement. Readers are encouraged to note the different shadings in the theories and definitions of these three quality improvement experts.

Although these thoughts were not formulated specifically for health care, the concepts are essential to understand if health care providers, including solo practitioners and practitioners who are part of organizations, are to meet the quality challenge facing health care today.

W. Edwards Deming[2]

W. Edwards Deming is one of the quality consultants credited with revolutionizing Japanese industry and helping it to achieve an unprecedented level of quality and productivity.[3] Deming's approach to quality is encapsulated in his famous 14 points for management. These 14 points are outlined in Table 1 and discussed in more detail below. Some are more clearly relevant to health care than others, but all are important.

Point 1: *Create constancy of purpose toward improvement of product and service.* The aim of this point, says Deming, is "to become competitive..., to stay in business, and to provide jobs." To fulfill this aim, organizations must, while not ignoring the "problems of today" such as budget, employment, and public relations, deal with the more challenging "problems of tomorrow." Coping with future problems requires the constancy of purpose Deming stresses in this point. This constancy of purpose entails not allowing the desire for immediate profit to hurt the organization's long-term improvement and competitiveness. For long-term improvement to occur, management must *innovate* by allocating resources for long-term planning, must *put resources into research and education,* and must *constantly improve design of product and service.* Regarding constant improvement, Deming reminds management that "this obligation never ceases." These actions are as difficult and as essential in the health care field as they are in industry.

Point 2: *Adopt the new philosophy.* The new philosophy

Deming refers to is, of course, quality improvement as practiced in Japan. Adopting this philosophy means stopping the practices into which American industry has fallen:

> We can no longer tolerate commonly accepted levels of mistakes, defects, material not suited for the job, people on the job that do not know what the job is and are afraid to ask, handling damage, antiquated methods of training on the job, inadequate and ineffective supervision, management not rooted in the company, job hopping in management...[2]

Deming does not direct his challenge only to management, but states government must remove obstacles to American industry's competitive position.

Point 3: *Cease dependence on inspection to achieve quality.* Inspection implies rework. It implies that defects will occur and will need to be repaired. Although inspection may be necessary for safety and accuracy, especially in certain very complex processes and products, reliance on inspection means that attention is not focused on improvement to make the outcome right the first time. "Inspection does not improve quality, nor guarantee quality. Inspection is too late."

Point 4: *End the practice of awarding business on the basis of price tag.* Price does not indicate quality; when the item purchased is not of high quality, high costs (such as maintenance and frequent replacement) can result. Deming suggests long-term relationships with single vendors will elicit loyalty, trust, and, in the long run, lower costs.

Point 5: *Improve constantly and forever the system of production and service.* One way to explain this point is to say what it does *not* mean. It does not mean "putting out fires," that is, solving immediate problems as they crop up. Rather, it means an ongoing commitment to assure quality is "built in at the design stage" or that all existing processes are continually studied and revised to improve their outputs. How is this improvement done? Not, Deming says, by simply allocating money for quality. Knowledge is key. The better understanding management and others have of the processes employed, the more effective change will be. Using reliable statistical methods to study processes is also necessary and will be discussed in Chapter Four.

Point 6: *Institute training on the job.* Deming stresses two kinds of training. First, management must be trained in the complete function of the organization and in the concepts of quality improvement, especially a focus on reducing vari-

---

W. EDWARDS DEMING'S 14 POINTS FOR MANAGEMENT*

1. Create constancy of purpose toward improvement of product and service.

2. Adopt the new philosophy.

3. Cease dependence on inspection to achieve quality.

4. End the practice of awarding business on the basis of price tag.

5. Improve constantly and forever the system of production and service.

6. Institute training on the job.

7. Institute leadership.

8. Drive out fear, so that everyone may work effectively for the company.

9. Break down barriers between departments.

10. Eliminate slogans, exhortations, and targets for the work force.

11. Eliminate numerical quotas and management by objective.

12. Remove barriers to pride of workmanship.

13. Institute a vigorous program of education and self-improvement.

14. Put everybody in the organization to work to accomplish the transformation.

Sources: Deming WE: Out of the Crisis. Cambridge, MA: Massachusetts Institute of Technology, 1986, pp 23-24; Walton M: The Deming Management Method. New York: Dodd, Mead & Company, 1986, pp 55-88.

Table 1

---

ation rather than on meeting specifications. Second, appropriate training and placement for staff will assure their rich talents are not squandered. Appropriate training for staff, and management, includes (a) assuring there *is* training, (b) making sure the means of training is effective (for example, eliminating inscrutable written instructions), and (c) ending the practice of having staff trained by other staff who, themselves, may have acquired bad habits because of poor training. Training should be ongoing while there is evidence it is helpful, and training should occur when circumstances require it, for example, when new equipment is put into use. Continuing education is, of course, a part of the culture in health care. That education should include the tenets of quality improvement and statistical quality control.

Point 7: Institute leadership. Management must, Deming says, not supervise but lead. To do this, management must "remove barriers that make it impossible for the hourly worker to do his [or her] job with pride of workmanship"; they also must intimately know the work they supervise. To lead, management also must not treat every problem as a fire to be put out, but must look toward system improvement. Finally, leaders should not fall into numerical fallacies, especially the notion that all workers should meet the average. In fact, not everyone can be above average; *some must always be below.* "The important problem is...who is statistically out of line and in need of help."

Point 8: Drive out fear. "No one can put in his best performance unless he feels secure." Fear is inherent in the bad-apple approach to quality and in the perception that quality is something imposed by outside forces peering over the shoulder of each member of the organization. "A common denominator of fear in any form, anywhere, is loss from impaired performance and padded figures." In health care, reticence to communicate problems because of fear, or "padding figures" because of fear, can have deadly consequences.

Point 9: Break down barriers between departments. The structure of an organization can work against quality improvement; lack of communication between departments and services can impede improvement and cause problems. In health care, this is especially true. The coordination of, for example, nursing, anesthesia, surgery, and post-anesthesia care are crucial for any surgical procedure. For another example, communication between professional and administrative staff is essential when contemplating equipment purchase or changes in procedures. In addition, the process by which systems are studied and improved requires close cooperation of all involved parties, no matter in what department or service each may work. Removing such barriers can mean a change in the culture of an organization.

Point 10: Eliminate slogans, exhortations, and targets for the work force. Here, Deming emphasizes that such tactics are meaningless without a plan to back them up. Also, they generate frustration by asking a worker to improve without providing the necessary means to do that.

Point 11: Eliminate numerical quotas and management by

W. EDWARDS DEMING'S SEVEN "DEADLY DISEASES"*

1. Lack of constancy of purpose to plan product and service that will have a market and keep the company in business, and provide jobs.

2. Emphasis on short-term profits: short-term thinking (just the opposite from constancy of purpose to stay in business), fed by fear of unfriendly takeover, and by push from bankers and owners for dividends.

3. Evaluation of performance, merit rating, or annual review.

4. Mobility of management; job hopping.

5. Management by use only of visible figures, with little or no consideration of figures that are unknown or unknowable.

6. Excessive medical costs.

7. Excessive costs of liability, swelled by lawyers who work on contingency fees.

*Source: Deming WE: Out of the Crisis. Cambridge, MA: Massachusetts Institute of Technology, 1986, pp 97-98.

Table 2

---

objective. "Rates for production are often set to accommodate the average worker. Naturally, half of them are above average, and half below.... The result is loss, chaos, dissatisfaction, and turnover. Some rates are set for the achiever, which is even worse." Quotas for management are equally problematic. Often they are not accompanied by plans, and if the system itself is not stable, a goal is meaningless.

Point 12: Remove barriers to pride of workmanship. Deming lists several specific barriers. One, he says, is the annual performance evaluation linked to a pay increase for people on salary. Such a system "focuses on the end product, at the end of the stream, not on leadership to help people." The effect is fear and self-preservation, not action to improve the organization. A barrier to staff pride is the sense that they are a commodity, the sense that they are powerless to communicate their ideas and knowledge to management, and the sense that they do not know what is expected of them. Quick-fix solutions to these barriers will not work; management must demonstrate over a period of time that they will take action to improve systems, that they are not engaged on a continuing hunt for bad apples, and that they are committed to the long-term survival and improvement of the organization.

Point 13: Institute a vigorous program of education and self-improvement. As stated under point 6, ongoing education of the sort practiced in the health care field is essential to make the most of talented people. In addition, as the organization changes as a result of quality improvement activities, re-education will be necessary to help people adapt to the changing environment.

Point 14: Put everybody in the organization to work to accomplish the transformation. Mary Walton, in her book The Deming Management Method, summarizes point 14 this way:

Management will have to organize itself as a team to advance the 13 other points. A statistical consultant will be required. Every employee of the company, including the managers, should acquire a precise idea of how to improve quality continually. The initiative must come from management.[3]

Deming emphasizes that the change will take place in stages, over time, and suggests specific actions to facilitate change. These will be introduced in Chapter Four, which deals extensively with implementation of quality improvement principles and activities.

Finally, Deming has also formulated what he calls the "seven deadly diseases" afflicting many organizations. These are listed in Table 2.

Joseph M. Juran[4]

For more than four decades, Joseph M. Juran has been conducting seminars and other training on quality management. He was one of the quality consultants credited with fueling the quality revolution in Japan. Through the Juran Institute, he continues to conduct open seminars and in-house seminars for managers throughout the world.

To condense Juran's extensive writings, this section will focus on his definition of quality and on the widely used Juran Trilogy.

Definition of quality. Juran suggests quality has a dual meaning. In one sense, quality refers to freedom from deficiencies, or, in more realistic terms, the error rate. In another sense, quality refers to product features, "a property... possessed by a product that is intended to meet certain customers' needs and thereby provide customer satisfac-

---

JOSEPH M. JURAN'S DEFINITION OF QUALITY

Product Features that Meet Customer Needs
Higher quality enables companies to:
- Increase customer satisfaction
- Make products salable
- Meet competition
- Increase market share
- Provide sales income
- Secure premium prices

The major effect is on sales
Usually, higher quality costs more

Freedom From Deficiencies
Higher quality enables companies to:
- Reduce error rates
- Reduce rework, waste
- Reduce field failures, warranty charges
- Reduce inspection, test shortens time to put new products onthe market
- Increase yields, capacity
- Improve delivery performance

Major effect is on costs
Usually higher quality costs less

Source: Juran JM: Juran on Leadership for Quality. New York, The Free Press, 1989. Used with permission.

Table 3

---

tion." Table 3 lists some aspects of each of these definitions of quality. Briefly, reduced deficiencies result in reduced rework, reduced need for inspection, and reduced customer dissatisfaction. Reduced deficiencies tend to lower costs. High quality in terms of product features, on the other hand, makes products appealing to consumers, increases sales, increases competitiveness, and often increases costs. This distinction is especially applicable to health care.

According to Juran, these two aspects of quality are not opposites. To satisfy customers, a product must both have the features they desire and be as free from deficiencies as possible. One or the other, alone, does not constitute high quality.

The short definition of quality that Juran says is widely accepted is "fitness for use." This definition embodies both the freedom-from-deficiencies and the product-features approaches to quality. Juran suggests that companies establish clear definitions of quality and of terms such as product, product features, and customer.

The Juran Trilogy. Juran's trilogy offers three processes by which managers maintain and improve quality:

1. Quality planning;
2. Quality control; and
3. Quality improvement.

The relationship and function of these three processes is depicted in Figure 2 and summarized in the following paragraphs.

Quality planning is the means by which upper managers

- Determine who the customers are;
- Determine the needs of the customers;
- Develop product features that respond to customers' needs;
- Develop processes able to produce the product features; and
- Transfer the plans to the operating forces.

Quality planning involves building quality into the processes and the product—quality in terms of freedom from deficiencies and desirability of product features.

Quality control refers to "'holding the status quo': keeping a planned process in its planned state so that it remains able to meet the operating goals." Although quality planning may have designed a stable process, quality control recognizes that a host of forces may affect the process. Quality control involves

- evaluating actual performance;
- comparing actual performance to goals; and
- taking action on the differences.

Juran describes the "feedback loop" by which quality control takes place (see Figure 3). In this loop, the process includes a "sensor," which evaluates performance. The sensor passes this information on to an "umpire," who also knows the established goal for the process. The umpire "compares actual performance to the goal" to determine whether "the difference warrants action." If so, the umpire forwards this message to the "actuator," who "makes the changes needed to bring performance into line with goals."

Juran defines *quality improvement* as "the organized creation of beneficial change" and "the attainment of unprecedented levels of performance." He refers to this as "breakthrough." In Figure 2, the quality improvement stage of the trilogy is illustrated by a significant improvement in operations, mov-

THE QUALITY TRILOGY

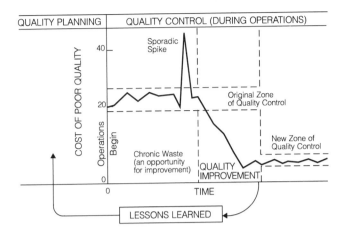

Figure 2
Joseph M. Juran's "Quality trilogy" quality planning, quality control, and quality improvement. Reprinted with permission from: Juran JM: Juran on Leadership for Quality. New York: The Free Press, 1989.

ing the "zone of quality control" to a new level.

Enacting quality improvement is a complex task. It involves all the elements shown in Table 4, including

- establishing the necessary infrastructure;
- identifying the specific improvement projects;
- establishing a team for each project;
- providing the resources, motivation, and training for the teams to diagnose the causes, establish or stimulate a remedy, and establish controls to hold the gains.

THE FEEDBACK LOOP

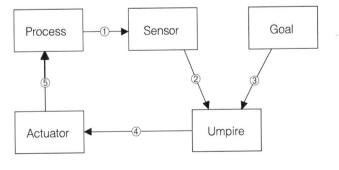

Figure 3
This diagram illustrates the "feedback loop" through which quality control is carried out. Reprinted with permission from: Juran JM: Juran on Leadership for Quality. New York: The Free Press, 1989.

Juran stresses that quality improvement "takes place project by project." Diagnosing and remedying quality deficiencies does require an investment, but Juran offers strong evidence that the "return on investment is among the highest available to managers." Juran also offers detailed information on how to establish a quality council, select projects, establish teams, and take action.

Quality improvement is an ongoing process that should have high priority among upper management. "Typically," Juran writes, "it has taken several years to establish quality improvement as a continuing, integral part of a company's business plan."

Philip B. Crosby[5]

Philip B. Crosby is a widely respected quality consultant. He rose from line inspector of ITT to corporate vice president, giving him a unique look at quality from various points of view. His books include Quality Is Free, The Art of Getting Your Own Sweet Way, and Quality Without Tears. Like Deming, Crosby emphasizes the importance of systems knowledge and improvement, the drawbacks of inspection, and the need for statistical quality control. The following are Crosby's "Four Absolutes":

The first absolute: The definition of quality is conformance to requirements. Crosby says the key to quality improvement is to "do it right the first time." He has assigned an acronym to this concept: DIRFT. To assure everyone will DIRFT, management must "(1) establish the requirements that employees are to meet, (2) supply the wherewithal that the employees need in order to meet those requirements, and (3) spend all its time encouraging and helping the employees to meet those requirements." The first condition is to define quality by establishing requirements. Conforming to these specific requirements is the goal; it is quality. Without such requirements, even skilled, creative staff and insightful managers cannot DIRFT because they do not know what the "it" is that they are supposed to do right. The second two conditions (supplying the wherewithal and spending time encouraging and helping) are other means by which management demonstrates its commitment to quality.

The second absolute: The system of quality is prevention. This absolute stresses the futility of relying solely on after-the-fact methods to improve quality. These encourage staff to find ways around, rather than solve, the difficulties. For example, a company may order more of a certain part than is needed, because the part has a known level of defects. Or a data system known to be problematic may be supplemented by a backup system. Or staff may be added to do rework

---

**INTERRELATION OF THE ELEMENTS OF QUALITY IMPROVEMENT
AS DESCRIBED BY JOSEPH M. JURAN**

Mobilizing for Quality Improvement

Establish quality council
Statement of responsibilities
Improvement policies, goals

Establish Infrastructure	Projects Collectively	Projects Individually
Subcouncils	Srategic improvement goals	Nomination
Director of quality	Deployment	Screening
Quality-improvement managers	Projects	Selection
Sponsors, champions	Resources	Mission statements
Facilitators	Progress review	Project teams
Structured improvement process	Recognition	Life cycle of a project:
Training: methods: tools	Rewards	diagnosis; remedy; cloning

Source: Juran JM: Juran on Leadership for Quality. New York: The Free Press, 1989. Used with permission.

Table 4

resulting from a system problem. Crosby suggests the waste involved in such solutions is "incredible." A more effective solution is prevention. Prevention is improving the process so the errors or problems don't occur in the first place. Prevention is impossible, however, without a clear understanding of the process in question. An important tool for prevention is statistical quality control. This method helps staff and management know when a process is out of control. Of course, once data show a process is out of control, action must be taken to improve it. A policy of prevention is futile if data showing performance out of the control limits are routinely ignored.

The third absolute: The performance standard is zero defects. Beyond setting requirements, Crosby stresses that requirements must always be met. When a company does not demonstrate that requirements must always be met, it "encourages people not to do everything right.... No one knows exactly what will or won't occur." A company cannot afford to send this message and should avoid setting acceptable levels of nonconformity or other means to "help their people not meet the requirements." Crosby emphasizes, "The performance standard must be 'zero defects,' not 'that's close enough.'"

The fourth absolute: The measurement of quality is the price of nonconformance. The cost of quality is not simply the cost of defects. The "price of nonconformance" includes "all expenses involved in doing things wrong": correcting paperwork, correcting processes, correcting products or services, paying claims. In service companies, the cost of nonconformance is 35% of operating costs. The price of conformance, on the other hand, is a far lower figure. The price of conformance is "what is necessary to spend to make things come out right." Crosby encourages companies to keep track of the cost of quality, because this is a persuasive way to measure quality and to demonstrate the value of quality improvement.

Beyond these four absolutes, Crosby proposes a vaccine

PROFILE OF A QUALITY-TROUBLED COMPANY

Characteristic	That's us all the way	Some is true	We're not like that
1. Our services and/or products normally contain waivers, deviations, and other indications of their not conforming to requirements.			
2. We have a "fix it" oriented field service and/or dealer organization.			
3. Our employees do not know what management wants from them concerning quality.			
4. Management does not know what the piece of performance really is.			
5. Management believes that quality is a problem caused by something other than management action.			
	5 points	3 points	1 point

Point count condition

21 - 25 Critical: Needs intensive care immediately.
16 - 20 Guarded: Needs life support system hookup.
11 - 15 Resting: Needs medication and attention.
 6 - 10 Healing: Needs regular checkup.
     5 Whole: Needs counseling.

Figure 4
This figure shows common characteristics of organizations needing a quality-improvement program.
Reprinted with permission from Crosby PB: Quality Without Tears. New York: McGraw-Hill Book Company, 1984, p 4.

THE CROSBY VACCINATION SERUM INGREDIENTS*

Integrity

A. The chief executive officer is dedicated to having the customer receive what is promised, believes that the company will prosper only when all employees feel the same way, and is determined that neither customers nor employees will be hassled.

B. The chief operating officer believes that management performance is a complete function requiring that quality be "first among equals"—schedule and cost.

C. The senior executives, who report to those in A and B, take requirements so seriously that they can't stand deviations.

D. The managers, who work for the senior executives, know that the future rests with their ability to get things done through people—right the first time.

E. The professional employees know that the accuracy and completeness of their work determines the effectiveness of the entire work force.

F. The employees as a whole recognize that their individual commitment to the integrity of requirements is what makes the company sound.

Systems

A. The quality management function is dedicated to measuring conformance to requirements and reporting any differences accurately.

B. The quality education system (QES) ensures that all employees of the company have a common language of quality and understand their personal roles in causing quality to be routine.

C. The financial method of measuring nonconformance and conformance costs is used to evaluate processes.

D. The use of the company's services or products by customers is measured and reported in a manner that causes corrective action to occur.

E. The companywide emphasis on defect prevention serves as a base for continual review and planning that utilizes current and past experience to keep the past from repeating itself.

Communications

A. Information about the progress of quality improvement and achievement actions is continually supplied to all employees.

B. Recognition programs applicable to all levels of responsibility are a part of normal operations.

C. Each person in the company can, with very little effort, identify error, waste, opportunity, or any other concern to top management quickly—and receive an immediate answer.

D. Each management status meeting begins with a factual and financial review of quality.

Operations

A. Suppliers are educated and supported in order to ensure that they will deliver services and products that are dependable and on time.

B. Procedures, products, and systems are qualified and proven prior to implementation and then continually examined and officially modified when the opportunity for improvement is seen.

C. Training is a routine activity for all tasks and is particularly integrated into new processes and procedures.

Policies

A. The policies on quality are clear and unambiguous.

B. The quality function reports on the same level as those functions that are being measured and has complete freedom of activity.

C. Advertising and all external communications must be completely in compliance with the requirements that the products and services must meet.

Source: Crosby PB: Quality Without Tears. New York: McGraw-Hill, 1984, pp 8-9. Used with permission.

Table 5

to provide "antibodies that will prevent hassle." This "quality vaccine" is a clear picture of the characteristics of an organization that fulfills the principles of quality improvement. To administer this vaccine, management must have determination to implement quality improvement, must educate all employees in quality improvement, and must be dedicated to the long process of implementing quality improvement (rather than looking for a quick fix). Table 5 presents the ingredients of Crosby's "quality vaccine."

Crosby has also developed a pithy chart used to ascertain whether an organization suffers from the symptoms of trouble that make his vaccine necessary. This chart is reprinted in Figure 4.

QUALITY IMPROVEMENT AND HEALTH CARE

Based on the ideas and experiences of these experts, the following summary of quality improvement principles can be put forward: Quality improvement involves deemphasizing inspection and emphasizing overall improvement by using reliable methods to study processes, by removing barriers to cooperation, by taking necessary actions to improve processes, and by fostering a constructive organizationwide commitment to improvement.

Does this industry-based concept of quality improvement apply to health care? Many experts believe the answer is yes, although that affirmative answer is usually accompanied by cautions. Chapter Three will describe how quality improvement can be used in health care, along with the potential difficulties and how to cope with them. Chapter Five will then outline steps health care organizations can take to put quality improvement into action.

REFERENCES
1. Berwick DM: Curing Health Care, New Strategies for Quality Improvement. San Francisco: Jossey-Bass Publishers, 1990.
2. Deming WE: Out of the Crisis. Cambridge, MA: Massachusetts Institute of Technology, 1986.
3. Walton M: The Deming Management Method. New York: Dodd, Mead & Company, 1986.
4. Juran JM: Juran on Leadership for Quality. New York: The Free Press, 1989.
5. Crosby PB: Quality Without Tears. New York: McGraw-Hill, 1984.

Chapter Three

QUALITY IMPROVEMENT IN HEALTH CARE

A test result lost, a specialist who cannot be reached, a missing requisition, a misinterpreted order, duplicate paperwork, a vanished record, a long wait for the CT scan, an unreliable on-call system—these are all-too-familiar examples of waste, rework, complexity, and error in the doctor's daily life.... For the average doctor, quality fails when systems fail.[1]

Can quality improvement techniques be applied to health care? This was the primary question posed by the National Demonstration Project on Quality Improvement in Health Care, which coupled industrial quality experts with teams from 21 health care organizations. The results of this project are reported in the book Curing Health Care:

> One by one, these pioneer teams reported back simple, elegant stories of successful application of the basic tools that illuminate processes and reveal causes of variation: process flow diagrams..., run charts, scatter plots, and control charts....The result was often new insights into old and familiar problems.
>
> In these project reports, we read several times that, through the use of the tools supplied by the quality control experts, "We saw things in a new and different way..." Armed by new understandings, the project teams were able to design interventions guided by process knowledge; they were not flying blind anymore.[2]

Among the conclusions of this project is that "Quality improvement tools can work in health care."[2] The Joint Commission concurs. A top-level commitment to quality, a non-punitive environment, education in quality improvement techniques, attention to opportunities to improve systems, and commitment of resources to carry out ongoing improvement all

can result in improved understanding of quality, desire to improve quality, and actual quality improvement.

Along with these attractions of quality improvement in health care, several difficulties present themselves. For example, much of the industry-focused quality improvement literature speaks of "defects" and "standards" that apply to the "product." In health care, the "product" is not as easily described in such objective terms. No two patients are the same; age, comorbidities, and other factors affect treatment and outcomes. This lack of uniformity makes measuring quality and determining which actions will improve it something less than an exact science. (Approaches to objectively assessing and improving health care quality are discussed in Chapter Five. Readers are also referred to the Primer on Indicator Development and Application, available from the Joint Commission.)

Another potential problem is acquiring the management commitment to quality improvement—in particular, the investment of time and money. Experience in industries and service organizations suggests that, ultimately, quality improvement will save money. However, health care organizations are just beginning to implement quality improvement; the implementation process can be protracted, and savings will likely not be immediate. Governing boards, administrative leaders, and clinical leaders must acknowledge the *need* for quality improvement and understand its concepts to be committed to its implementation.

Along with management commitment, physician involvement is critical to quality improvement. Physician expertise will be necessary to assess and improve clinical care, as well as to signal that quality improvement is an organizationwide effort, not merely the duty of a single department or the latest fad. Physician involvement may not, however, be easy to come by. Traditionally, physicians have had a great deal of autonomy within the hospital, which may work against the team effort implicit in quality improvement. Physicians who are not full-time hospital employees may require extra incentives to participate. Also, past resistance to quality assurance (the perception of its punitive nature, the perception that it encouraged "cookbook medicine") could carry over to quality improvement.

Although it is tempting to present quality improvement as a panacea, at this early stage, it is wise to temper the enthusiasm with the acknowledgment that much remains to be learned as health care organizations begin the transition to quality improvement.

ELEMENTS OF QUALITY IMPROVEMENT IN HEALTH CARE

Having outlined the principles of quality improvement as it applies to industry, this chapter shows how those principles apply to health care. Drawing from the industrial models discussed in Chapter Two, from quality improvement theorists and practitioners in and out of health care, and from the research efforts of the Joint Commission's Agenda for Change, the following elements of quality improvement in health care emerge:

- Quality is a central priority for the organization.
- The organization leaders are knowledgeable in, committed to, and involved in quality improvement.
- Quality improvement efforts focus on functions and processes.
- The organization uses reliable statistical methods to measure performance of both processes and outcomes.
- All staff in the organization participate and cooperate in the quality improvement effort. All barriers to cooperation are removed and dialogue between "customers" and "suppliers" is encouraged.
- The organization evinces a spirit of respect and support, in which leaders assume those providing care are capable and will welcome the chance to improve their effectiveness by removing procedural defects that impede quality.

The next sections describe these elements in more depth.

Quality as a Central Priority

The experts agree that quality improvement cannot be effective without a clear indication that it is a central priority in the organization. This indication must come from the leaders in the form of a quality-focused mission statement along with planning and support for daily activities designed to improve quality.

Mission and vision statement. A mission statement indicates why an organization exists. A vision statement describes what the organization wishes to be, including its view of itself, and its relationship to those it serves. The self-definition inherent in drafting mission and vision statements can be enlightening: the problems of the moment fall away and reveal the vision for tomorrow. Mission and vision statements that place quality in the forefront of organizational commitments send a strong message to leaders, staff, and the public.

Daily activities. Naturally, a mission statement that does not translate into action quickly becomes a dusty document, more evidence of wasted effort and paper. The organization leaders must back up their defined commitment to quality with "additional investments in managerial time, capital, and technical expertise";[1] with innovation, research, education, continuous improvement, and knowledge of customers;[3] and with integrity, systems, communications, operations, and policies.[3]

Thus, the quality commitment must be demonstrated by investment in time, funds, education, and research; by a clear plan composed of effective policies and procedures; by department heads, administrators, and other leaders who enact the plan to carry out the mission and realize the vision.

Leaders' Involvement

Leaders play a key role in fostering quality improvement. "The job of management," Deming says, "is not supervision, but leadership."[3] To lead in quality improvement, the responsible individuals must have knowledge about and be actively involved in quality.

Knowledge. Knowledge of the concepts and techniques of quality improvement is essential if the activities are to be effective. Without this knowledge, the leaders' actions become an empty formality, and the leaders cannot make informed decisions about effectiveness or the need to improve activities.

Such knowledge is by no means a given. Evolving thinking about quality in health care can leave many professionals without key information on how quality improvement is best carried out. In addition, some basic knowledge of statistical techniques and ways data are organized are required if the leaders are to understand and interpret findings.

A key to quality improvement is improving processes. Leaders must be knowledgeable about the processes and systems in the organization to oversee their improvement.

Involvement. An important part of the leaders' role is finding the right people for the right jobs. But the leaders also should be actively involved in quality improvement. They should help set priorities for improvement, receive reports on activities, and react to those reports by, as appropriate, helping to interpret data or formulate necessary actions, approving necessary actions, and reevaluating priorities for monitoring. Quality improvement principles should also be applied to the work the leaders themselves perform.

Focus on Processes

Hospital staff are well aware of difficulties in scheduling, transferring information, dispensing medications, and many other facets of hospital operation.[1] Such widespread difficulties are not often the fault of incompetent individuals; rather, flaws built into these processes prevent competent individuals from providing care and service as well as they would like. Searching for individuals not performing up to par—the "bad apples"—is commonly known as "quality by inspection." This approach to quality has serious detriments.

First, it creates an environment of fear, defensiveness, and isolation. Staff who believe their hands will be slapped for errors will seldom report problems (whether "errors" or not); thus, data are distorted and opportunities for improvement concealed. In such an environment, the whole notion of quality is inexorably linked to negation. On a larger scale, the current health care environment lends itself to quality by inspection, the search for bad apples. External reviewers and regulators are perceived as threatening forces, requiring data that may be used against the hospital. Even popular movies and television programs focus on the mishaps or avarice of individual practitioners.

Second, inspection has a negligible effect on quality. Certainly, if a specific problem practitioner is identified, actions should be taken, and presumably his or her errors will no longer crop up on quality assurance reports. But Deming calls this "putting out fires," finding problems "too late."[3] And Crosby states, "Appraisal is an expensive and unreliable way of getting quality. Checking and sorting and evaluating only sift what is done. What has to happen is prevention. The error that does not exist cannot be missed."[4]

If an individual is identified and his or her problem solved,

that does not solve the broader problems of misscheduled operating rooms and equipment, medication errors, incomplete patient records, and so forth; in short, the nagging process difficulties that compose everyday life in a health care institution will continue after the fire is put out. The norm of performance will be all but unchanged.

A more productive goal would be to *raise the norm of performance*. Raising the norm is achieved by

- studying and understanding the complex processes that contribute to care;
- measuring performance of processes and their outcomes using valid statistical methods; and
- taking action to improve the way processes are designed and carried out.

Although it will always be important to assess the competence and performance of individuals providing care, broader improvement is possible by improving processes.

This focus on process does not mean that outcomes are no longer a concern. The study and understanding of processes will reveal which processes and steps in the processes are most closely linked to important outcomes. Thus, improved processes should result in improved outcomes. Outcomes may be monitored to direct attention to any process that needs revision to improve the outcome.

Reliable Statistical Methods

Accurate data are important ingredients of quality improvement. These data are acquired using the tested techniques of statistical quality control. Without these methods, unsystematic data collection and subjective evaluation of care can render the quality improvement activities futile. Philip Crosby describes statistical quality control this way:

> [Statistical quality control] is made out to be very complicated and difficult to do, but there really isn't that much to it. It is a very effective, easy-to-understand tool. The people who make up the charts for the variables and teach the measurement techniques have to be skilled, but everyone else only has to learn to understand a few things.
>
> The charts are made up with an upper and lower limit representing the "tolerance" of the process. Each measurement is recorded by a dot on the chart. If a dot is within the lines, keep running. If the dots are heading outside the lines, do something. If a dot is over the line, shut down. That is all there is to it.[4]

The tools of statistical quality control, including cause-and-effect diagrams, flow charts, pareto charts, run charts, histograms, scatter diagrams, and control charts will be discussed in the next chapter. For now, it is enough simply to note the importance of reliable data to quality improvement.

Cooperative Effort

Quality must be the responsibility of everyone in the organization. The governing body, management, clinical staff, and support staff all must be involved in the effort, whether by overseeing and designing activities, participating in quality improvement teams, collecting data, or striving to improve their own performance.

To make this widespread involvement meaningful, real cooperation must exist among health care professionals, especially across perceived barriers such as departmental lines. Many processes in the hospital require participation of several departments or services, and a failure to communicate and coordinate among departments can interfere with effective interaction between the "customers" and "suppliers" within the organization. To improve the "hand offs" of care, barriers to cooperation must be removed.

In addition, it is essential that physicians participate in quality improvement. Donald Berwick, who has written extensively about quality improvement in health care, says that "physicians...seem to have difficulty seeing themselves as participants in processes, rather than as lone agents of success or failure."[1] Cultural divisions and barriers are as important to remove as structural ones; indeed, they must be removed if significant improvement is to be seen.

A Spirit of Respect and Support

Finally, quality improvement requires "the belief that those involved in health care are genuinely committed to doing their best."[5] The system is doomed to failure if it carries over the negative connotations—justified or not—of quality assurance: that it is performed only to satisfy external forces, that its purpose is to identify and discipline individuals, that its rewards are difficult to discern, that organization leaders will not support the efforts.

A clear message must be communicated to the organization: management and quality improvement are here to help, not to slap wrists. The leaders will commit resources to reduce double-work, eliminate wasted effort, and improve communication so the organization's competent, caring, dedicated, hard-working staff can perform with the fewest obstructions.

FROM PRINCIPLES TO ACTION

The elements of quality improvement in health care discussed in this chapter are aptly summarized in these four points:

1. All key activities of an organization should further its mission. In health care, the central and sustaining mission is to meet the health care needs of patients in as efficient and effective a manner as possible.

2. Fulfillment of this mission requires a coordinated effort by everyone in the organization—the Board, management, clinical staff, and support staff.

3. The most direct and predictable route to cost-effective care is for individuals and operational groups in the organization to understand the key processes they engage in, to measure the efficiency and effectiveness of these processes, and to improve them whenever possible.

4. This search for constant improvement will be successful only if everyone adopts the belief that those involved in health care are genuinely committed to doing their best. We must never allow an impaired or incompetent colleague to harm patients, but while doing so, our *principal* challenge is to help *everyone* improve.[5]

Some means by which these elements of quality improvement can be put into action are implicit: attitude changes, investment, expertise, and so on. But questions about implementing quality improvement remain: How can an organization instill attitude changes? Where will the money for investments come from? How can an organization acquire the statistical expertise it needs? Another lingering question is what should be done with all the quality assurance activities health care organizations have been performing—monitoring and evaluation, drug usage evaluation, surgical case review, and so forth.

Chapter Four addresses how quality improvement can be implemented in a health care organization and how Joint Commission standards are changing to reflect this transition.

REFERENCES

1. Berwick DM: Continuous improvement as an ideal in health care. N Engl J Med 320(1): 53-56.

2. Berwick DM: Curing Health Care, New Strategies for Quality Improvement. San Francisco: Jossey-Bass Publishers, 1990.

3. Deming WE: Out of the Crisis. Cambridge, MA: Massachusetts Institute of Technology, 1986.

4. Crosby PB: Quality Without Tears. New York: McGraw-Hill, 1984.

5. Roberts JS and Schyve PS: From QA to QI: The views and role of the Joint Commission. The Quality Letter, May 1990.

Chapter Four

PUTTING QUALITY IMPROVEMENT INTO ACTION

Determination evolves when the members of a management team decide that they have had enough and are not going to take it any more. They recognize that their action is the only tool that will change the profile of the organization.[1]

With the principles of quality improvement and their application to health care in hand, the next question is how to implement quality improvement. Health care organizations embarking on the transition to quality improvement need an idea of the necessary steps, the possible barriers, and the time frame for implementation.

One way the Joint Commission can help facilitate the transition to quality improvement is through its standards. As outlined in Chapter One, Joint Commission standards are being revised and reorganized to allow and encourage the important growth quality improvement requires. This chapter explains those standards changes in depth, discusses possible barriers to quality improvement, and suggests the steps an organization can take to put quality improvement into action. Chapter Five follows up with specific assessment and improvement methods, including monitoring and evaluation.

JOINT COMMISSION STANDARDS

Joint Commission standards are changing to reflect the elements of quality improvement in health care. Historically, Joint Commission standards have been organized into department-specific chapters and have described the structures and processes related to quality of care. This approach has led to fragmentation of intent and duplication of the standards. In revising the standards, the Joint Commission has responded to hospital concerns expressed in focus group and feedback sessions to delete standards not specifically related to quality and those that appear redundant.

The major changes will include the following:

- The studied deletion of a number of predominantly structural standards requirements;
- The creation of new standards that emphasize the application of quality improvement concepts and shift the evaluation focus from individual departments to organizationwide performance; and
- The consolidation, recasting, and reorganization of all remaining standards into an accreditation manual format that directs attention to the performance of specified important functions of the organization.

The 1992 Standards

The 1992 Accreditation Manual for Hospitals (AMH) begins the transition to these objectives. Certain standards are revised to reduce or eliminate potential barriers for hospitals that are currently shifting to a quality improvement approach. In addition, the 1992 AMH has eliminated major portions of the standards that are not surveyed or that have little influence on patient outcomes. The 1992 AMH has also introduced standards that describe the characteristics of a process measurement and improvement system focused on continual enhancement in performance. Specific changes follow.

Quality assessment and improvement. In the 1992 AMH, the former "Quality Assurance" chapter is renamed "Quality Assessment and Improvement" and includes some significant revisions. First, the chapter includes a preamble that discusses the transition from quality assurance to quality improvement and explains that the standards are based on the principles of quality improvement.

Second, the preamble that formerly described the ten-step monitoring and evaluation process is deleted. Elsewhere, the standards pertaining to the monitoring and evaluation process have been clarified.

Third, barriers to organizationwide quality assessment and improvement have been removed. These barriers are the almost exclusive focus on clinical aspects of care, compartmentalization of quality activities according to hospital structure, focus on the performance of individuals more than on systems, and initiation of action only when a problem is identified.

Fourth, new standards QA.1 through QA.1.6 have been added; these address the roles of hospital leaders in ongoing quality improvement.

Fifth, the requirement to use monthly meetings of the clinical departments of the medical staff as the only acceptable mechanism to consider monitoring and evaluation findings has been deleted.

In addition, the phrase "quality assessment and improvement" has been substituted for "quality assurance." Also, the phrase "and appropriateness" has been eliminated from "monitoring and evaluating the quality and appropriateness of care" because contemporary definitions of quality include appropriateness as one of quality's components.

The revised 1992 quality assessment and improvement standards appear in Appendix A.

Medical staff monitoring. Revisions in three of the so-called medical staff monitoring functions have also been made in the 1992 standards. Specifically, the revised standards address the review of surgical and other invasive procedures, review of effective medication use, and review of blood and blood components. Traditionally, organizations have had difficulty fulfilling these standards, and some questions arose about their content. In an effort to improve these standards, revision has addressed three areas: sampling, subject of review, and primary focus on individuals.

The previous standards either specified or implied that review should include all cases and all practitioners. For surgical case review and blood usage review, the hospital was asked to review 100% of cases and demonstrate good performance before a smaller sample could be used. The revised standards clarify that such initial 100% review may not be necessary for high-frequency activities.

The subject of the review is also clarified by the proposed standards. The surgical and other invasive procedures review standards ask hospitals to focus on the "most important" categories of surgical and invasive procedures, and the blood and blood component review standards ask the hospital to focus on categories of blood and blood components, rather than each case. The medication use evaluation standards ask the hospital to focus on high-risk and problem-prone drugs, and those that are studied because they are used in particular illnesses under study.

Finally, these medical staff standards make it clear that the emphasis should be on the performance of key processes, not solely on review of individual practitioners.

These standards are reprinted in Appendix B.

The 1993 Standards

The 1993 AMH will reflect a continuation of the improvements made in the 1992 edition. While changes will be far less extensive, efforts to identify and consolidate "repetitive" standards will continue. For example, standards related to patient/family education and staff orientation. training, and education would have an organizationwide rather than a departmental application and would appear in a single section. In addition, standards will continue to be reviewed to evaluate their relevance to patient care quality and will be deleted or revised, as appropriate.

The 1994 Standards

An early draft of the 1994 quality assessment and improvement standards has been developed and helps show the direction this transition from quality assurance to quality improvement will take. The 1994 standards, which more fully incorporate principles and techniques that foster continuous improvement in performance and quality, are divided into five sections:

- *Leadership responsibility for quality improvement*—the leaders' responsibility to set expectations, develop plans, and implement procedures for quality improvement;
- *Techniques of quality improvement*—the process of ongoing monitoring, use of other feedback to trigger improvement, priority-setting for assessment and improvement, techniques of assessment and improvement, individuals'

activities in the process, and responsibility for the process;

- *Education and training*—the use of education in quality improvement, continuing education, human relationship training, and information support;
- *Communication and collaboration*—the mechanisms to facilitate communication among individuals and organizational components; and
- *Evaluation of effectiveness of quality improvement activities*—the need to regularly assess quality improvement activities, to use that assessment in planning, and to take actions based on the assessment.

These 1994 standards will continue the transition to quality improvement. Appendix C presents some ideas on the direction of future quality assessment and improvement standards and describes the kinds of issues that will be addressed in the 1994 standards.

DIFFICULTIES IN IMPLEMENTATION

As part of the standards-development process, an extensive field review of the 1992 standards was performed. Reviewers included medical staff presidents, chief executive officers, nurse executives, quality assurance professionals, medical record administrators, and many others. The results of this field review offer a penetrating list of the perceived difficulties of implementing quality improvement. Here are some of the issues identified:

Costs will increase. These increases were linked primarily to additional staffing and training, as well as to perceived need for improved information systems. These costs may be especially difficult for small and rural hospitals. One respondent commented,

It is likely that the increased involvement of leadership, coupled with the interdisciplinary/ interdepartmental nature of quality improvement, will require a greater time commitment on the part of management and clinical personnel than traditional quality assurance. In addition, education and training related to quality improvement methodologies will also result in increased cost to the institution. The need for more *sophisticated* information systems also will raise costs.

This concern about possible increased costs was frequently accompanied by a comment that indicated the cost would be worthwhile. For example, "[There will be] an increase in staff and training initially. In the long run, [however,]

costs will be offset by improved care, decreased lawsuits, and other 'goodwill benefits.'"

It *will be difficult to involve leadership*. Difficulties would arise, some respondents believed, in attempting to involve leaders in specific intra- and inter-departmental quality assessment and improvement activities. Although the standards ask that leaders assure the activities are carried out, rather than carry the activities out themselves, it is acknowledged that involvement of leadership (of the governing body, the medical staff, the nursing staff, and administration), as well as involvement of clinicians, will require a concerted effort.

An extended period of time will be required to implement quality improvement. Respondents to the field review believed it would take anywhere from seven months to five years to implement quality improvement as expressed in the new standards. A number of respondents mentioned that literature based on actual case studies indicates a three- to five-year time frame for the substantial change required to support continuous quality improvement.

Channels less formal than a field review have identified a number of other pressing concerns about implementing quality improvement. How will leaders and other staff learn about quality improvement? What are the statistical quality control techniques that are necessary? Will the Joint Commission still require monitoring and evaluation? In light of quality improvement, has monitoring and evaluation been futile? How, exactly, can departmental barriers be broken down?

These questions and concerns deserve a response. The following sections—cost, leadership, staff involvement, statistical quality control, and action plan—offer some answers. The question of specific monitoring, assessment, and improvement processes is large enough to require a chapter of its own—Chapter Five. In the aggregate, this material answers a central question about quality improvement: How do we get there?

COST

Cost is a sensitive concern to address. It is tempting to point toward future savings and say, "Don't worry, quality improvement will be worth every penny; it will pay for itself in the long run." True or not, organizations deserve to know how to deal with the cost of quality improvement now.

Organizations—especially small and rural hospitals—should keep in mind that neither the Joint Commission nor quality improvement requires *computerized* information systems. Organizations without automated systems certainly may consider implementing them. The savings in time over manual systems could be dramatic and realized within a reasonably limited time. However, this investment is not required. Small hospitals may very well find themselves able to adapt their present information systems to the techniques required for quality improvement. The same goes for other organizations: a radical overhaul of the information management system will likely not be necessary. What will be necessary is a new approach to how data can be used. This will be examined in the "Statistical Quality Control" section of this chapter.

Another potential fallacy is that a whole new army of education programs—time-consuming and expensive—will be necessary. Education is an ongoing process in health care organizations and takes many forms. For example, practitioners have already shown their willingness to regularly review the relevant literature, including literature pertaining to quality of care. Assuring that practitioners have articles and monographs that summarize the principles and techniques of quality improvement will go a long way toward providing the necessary education. Most organizations already make use of educational programs, including orientation, in-service programs, and outside programs, that address quality. It will only be necessary to make sure quality improvement is part of these programs, often replacing the emphasis on quality assurance. Many organizations make use of quality consultants and information management consultants. Make sure these consultants are well versed in quality improvement and that quality improvement is addressed in their assessments and suggestions.

Still, an investment will often be required. The Joint Commission cannot tell individual organizations where the money will come from. It can, however, stress the importance of what Philip Crosby would call "doing it right the first time." The "it," in this case, is quality improvement. A determined effort to change, the belief that change is necessary and possible, the commitment to the long-term well-being of the organization all require an investment in the people, equipment, and actions necessary to start the process in motion.

LEADERSHIP

Leadership knowledge, leadership commitment, leadership involvement—these qualities are stressed throughout

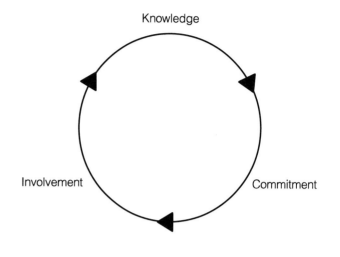

**CYCLE OF LEADERSHIP INVOLVEMENT
IN QUALITY IMPROVEMENT**

Figure 5

This diagram illustrates how leaders' knowledge about quality improvement will lead to a commitment to the program, and how that commitment will lead to involvement with its implementation. And as the program is implemented, further knowledge, commitment, and involvement will result.

the literature on quality improvement (including this book). The three are intertwined and cyclical. The diagram in Figure 5 depicts this cyclical nature. As leaders learn the tenets of quality improvement, they understand its importance in helping an organization to improve and survive. With this knowledge comes commitment to setting up such a program. Commitment to starting the program leads to involvement as the program is developed: involvement in assuring that staff are educated, any outside expertise is acquired, barriers to communication are removed, priorities for assessment and improvement are set, and systems and processes are understood. And when this stage of involvement is reached, knowledge increases again: the quality improvement program will direct attention to certain processes, stimulating their study. The leaders, by receiving reports on such activity and, when appropriate, approving the necessary actions, in turn acquire knowledge about the complex functions, systems, and processes in the organization and how they can be improved. This knowledge reenforces the commitment and increases the involvement.

But how is this cycle started? Philip Crosby says that

leaders must be fed up, must "have had enough" and be determined they are "not going to take it any more."[1] It is quite likely that some of the more odious aspects of the current climate in health care—pressure from external bodies and consumers, skyrocketing costs, personnel problems—have already provoked this attitude. Leaders, then, must know that continuous quality improvement is an option, a positive response to a seemingly untenable situation.

But who will tell them about quality improvement? The Joint Commission, for one. In its 1992 standards, and in those planned for 1994, the role of leadership in stimulating improvement is explicit. While hoping not to encourage the feeling that quality improvement is yet another hoop to be jumped through to please an external body, the Joint Commission nevertheless plays a role in building awareness, and its most potent means of communication is its standards. Accompanying the standards are publications, seminars, and consultation during surveys that support the importance of leadership involvement and other aspects of quality improvement.

Other important players in building awareness among leadership are the quality assurance or quality improvement professionals within health care organizations. These individuals are in a position to know more about quality improvement than perhaps anyone in the organization. Their responsibility, then, is to speak strongly to leaders on the subject, emphasizing potential benefits: improved environment (reduced fear, increased respect, increased cooperation), reduced costs in the short and long term, and increased quality.

Quality assurance/improvement professionals should also provide leaders with literature on the subject.

STAFF INVOLVEMENT

The cycle of staff involvement will likely be similar to that for leaders. The more they know about quality improvement, the more they will be committed to the process, the more they will be involved in the process, and so on. To promote initial knowledge about quality improvement, leaders must make the concept known: they must include it in orientation and training; they must circulate appropriate literature; they must demonstrate their commitment through investments and other actions. Without this demonstration from above, staff may well believe the promises of quality improvement to be empty, may see quality improvement as, in Deming's words, "instant pudding,"[2] or as the solution of the month.

Removing Communication Barriers

Staff involvement will also require removing communication barriers. Leaders can encourage interdepartmental communication by establishing a mechanism by which interdisciplinary teams are formed to address problems—and by giving those teams direction, assistance, and authority. (Deming calls such teams, when not backed by management commitment, a "cruel hoax."[2]) The organization can look for key areas that receive information affecting multiple departments (such as social work, patient/family relations, medical records) and provide those areas with an effective means to voice the findings and knowledge they have.

Health care organizations may encounter some difficulties in having individuals from different parts and different levels of the organization work together. Although these difficulties may never disappear completely, it is expected that the very process of quality improvement will reduce them. Interdisciplinary teams in which participation of all members is encouraged will give rise to mutual respect; study of the organization's complex processes will increase the awareness of individuals' and groups' interdependence; and improvement as a result of this cooperation will affirm the wisdom of working through any barriers to cooperation.

Another issue in staff involvement is gaining the cooperation of physicians. Again, the hospital culture may work against quality improvement here. Physicians tend to function independently and tend to see themselves as "lone agents of success or failure."[3] The following are a few methods leaders could consider in gaining physician support for and participation in quality improvement.[4]

Stress the benefits. Physicians (and other staff) may be suspicious if quality improvement is presented as a panacea, but they should be eager for a realistic chance to improve the efficiency and effectiveness in their daily professional lives, especially when that chance does not sound like a witch hunt. Would a physician like to stop waiting for a test result? Stop searching for lost information? Reduce the number of medication errors? The answer must be yes.

Make the program straightforward. Presenting, at the outset, an overly subtle, complex, and elaborate program, full of unnecessary refinement, will probably not gain favor with the medical staff. Such a program will be seen as time-consuming and potentially troublesome in the physician's busy schedule. A comprehensive yet concise proposal in common-sense terms will have the most chance of persuading physicians (and other staff) of its value.

Make it clear that quality improvement is not a witch hunt. One conception about quality assurance that hurt its acceptance with physicians was the sense that it hunted for individual practitioners not performing up to standards, documented that deviation, and meted out punishment. It should be clear from the outset that quality improvement is based on respect for practitioners and that it focuses on improving processes, not on punishing individuals.

Make it clear that quality improvement does not support "cookbook" medicine. Donald Berwick has some persuasive words about the "standards" of care that are often linked to "cookbook" medicine:

> Linked closely to the reliance on inspection to improve quality is the search for standards of care, which usually implies minimal thresholds of structure, process, or outcome above which one is safe from being labeled a Bad Apple. Quality-control engineers know that such floors rapidly become ceilings, and that a company that seeks merely to meet standards cannot achieve excellence.[3]

If systems are to be improved, however, they must be understood and measured. To do so, accurate delineations of process will be necessary, and physicians' input will be essential. Physicians should know that these delineations of process are not standards intended to stifle creativity and to be used against them.

Start at the top. One way organization leaders can effectively persuade practitioners of quality improvement's value is to start by getting key clinical leaders, especially department heads, to "buy into" the program. The immediacy of a strong message carried by respected clinicians will outweigh, say, a single memorandum from the chief executive officer.

STATISTICAL QUALITY CONTROL[5]

The importance of implementing statistical quality control has been mentioned several times in this publication. A thorough course in the techniques and implementation of statistical quality control is beyond the scope of this book; health care organizations should look to the experts for this instruction—through consultation, a staff expert, and the literature. What this section will attempt is to give readers a look at some charts and graphs used as tools in statistical quality control. (For more examples, see A Compendium of Forms, Tables, and Charts for Use in Monitoring and Evalu-

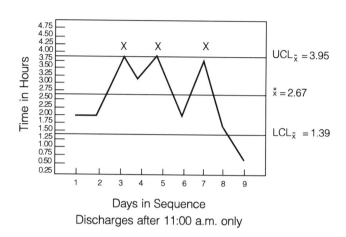

CONTROL CHART

Time in Hours / Days in Sequence

$UCL_{\bar{x}} = 3.95$

$\bar{\bar{x}} = 2.67$

$LCL_{\bar{x}} = 1.39$

Discharges after 11:00 a.m. only

Figure 6

Control chart showing admission process time from physician order to actual emergency room discharge. Reprinted with permission from: Berwick DM et al: Curing Health Care. San Francisco: Jossey-Bass Publishers, 1990.

ation, available from the Joint Commission. Some of these concepts are also addressed in Primer on Indicator Development and Application.)

Control Charts

A control chart shows performance data over a period of time to illustrate trends along with the average performance, the upper control limit, and the lower control limit. "These limits are not to be confused with specifications. The upper and lower control limits are determined by allowing a process to run untouched and then analyzing the results using a mathematical formula."[5] Figure 6 shows a control chart for admission process time from physician order to emergency room discharge. The line labeled $\bar{\bar{x}}$ indicates the average time; the UCL line is the upper control limit, and the LCL is the lower control limit.

The control chart shows variation in a process and whether that variation requires action. Performance moving toward a limit and performance outside the limit require action. Deming distinguishes between two kinds of variation. "Common cause" variations arise, as the name indicates, from small causes such as "minor variations in...ability, the clarity of procedures, the capability of...equipment, and so forth."[5] Common cause variations, then, generally pertain to systems. Solutions to such causes often require management action. "Special causes" are indicated by performance outside the control limits and are caused by such significant problems as equipment malfunction or an untrained employee.

One special value of a control chart is to help staff avoid looking at every random variation, because it acknowledges that some variation is to be expected.

Cause-and-Effect Diagrams

A cause-and-effect diagram illustrates a process as a set of causal factors and their consequences. Ideally, staff work together to formulate such a diagram before problems are noted or when a new process is being designed; it can also be used to help understand the cause of a problem in an existing system. Developing a cause-and-effect diagram helps shape staff's efforts to understand a process. Often it is helpful to put causes into some general categories, such as people, equipment, policies, and so forth. Figure 7 is a cause-and-effect diagram attempting to identify the various causes of postoperative infections.

CAUSE-AND-EFFECT DIAGRAM

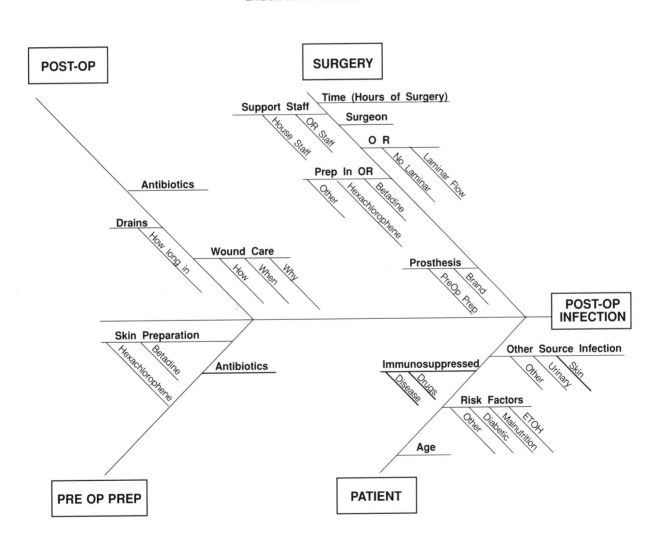

Source: Joint Commission: <u>How to Achieve Quality and Accreditation in a Hospital infection Control Program</u>.

Figure 7

This cause-and-effect diagram illustrates the complex causes that could lead to postoperative infection.

FLOWCHART

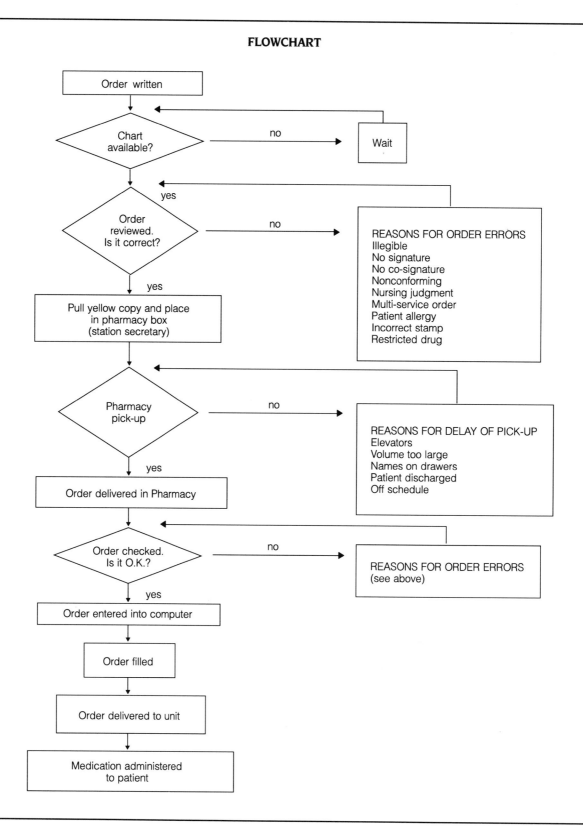

Figure 8

Flowchart depicting medication turnaround. Reprinted with permission from: Bader and Associates: Quality agenda: presenting quality improvement results to the board. The Quality Letter 3(4): 17-19, May 1991

PARETO CHART
Delayed discharges—September

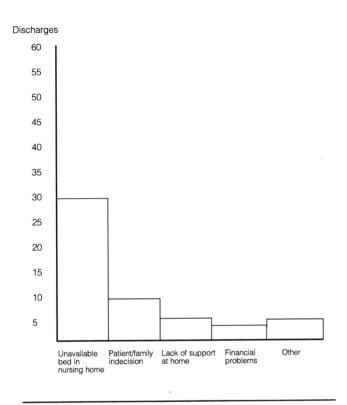

Figure 9

This figure shows how a pareto chart compares the causes of delayed discharge from a hospital. Staff may choose to follow up this chart with a chart comparing causes for unavailable beds.

Flowcharts

Flowcharts are well known in health care. They are often used to illustrate a decision-making process. Flowcharts present a series of steps and their sequels depending whether the preceding step takes place or not. In quality control, a flowchart can be used to understand a process and find problematic steps.

Figure 8 shows a flowchart describing how medication orders are processed along with reasons for delay.

Pareto Charts

"This chart is used to determine priorities. The pareto is sometimes described as a way to sort out the 'vital few' from the 'trivial many.'"[5] If, for example, a cause-and-effect diagram showed ten possible causes of delayed discharges, data would be collected to determine how frequently each cause comes into play. The pareto chart shown in Figure 9 illus-

RUN CHART

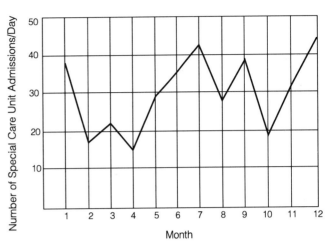

Figure 10

Run chart showing a hospital's number of special care unit admissions per day for one year. Source: Brassard M: The Memory Jogger: A Pocket Guide of Tools for Continuous Improvement, 2nd ed, Methuen, MA: Goal/QPC, 1988

trates the results of this data collection. Armed with such information, staff will know where to first focus their problem-solving actions.

Run Charts

Run charts are similar to control charts, but do not display the average or the control limits. In other words, a run chart simply displays performance over time to illustrate trends. A run chart could be useful to, for example, determine unit population to set staffing patterns. In the example in Figure 10, the run chart shows a hospital's number of special care unit admissions per day for one year.

Histograms

Histograms measure the rate and frequency of an occurrence. They can be used to measure productivity. A histogram could, for example, show the frequency at which medical records are completed within a given number of days after discharge. Figure 11 is a histogram depicting the response time from receipt of laboratory specimen on the evening shift. A histogram is used to examine common events and could be useful in formulating reasonable expectations for just how frequently the event occurs.

HISTOGRAM

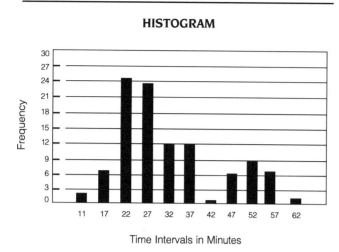

Time Intervals in Minutes

SCATTER CHART

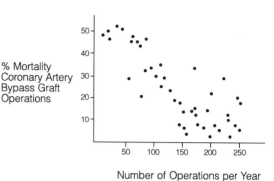

Number of Operations per Year

Figure 11

Histogram illustrating the response time from receipt of laboratory specimen on the evening shift. Reprinted with permission from: Berwick DM et al: Curing Health Care. San Francisco: Jossey-Bass Publishers, 1990

Figure 12

Scatter diagram comparing mortality rate for coronary artery bypass grafts and the number of operations performed per year. **Source:** adapted from: Merry MD: Total quality management for physicians: Translating the new paradigm. QRB 16(3): 103, Mar 1990. Used with permission.

Scatter Diagrams

Scatter diagrams show the relationship between two variables. If, for example, staff wanted to ascertain the relationship between mortality rate for coronary artery bypass graft operations and the number of operations performed per year, a scatter diagram such as that in Figure 12 could be created. Like the pareto chart, a scatter diagram provides staff data with which to evaluate cause-and-effect relationships.

The Value of Quality Control

Deming,[2,5] Ishikawa,[6] and other respected experts emphasize that quality control is a tool and not a substitute for a management commitment to quality improvement. Deming also warns against "proliferation of charts without purpose."[2] Statistical quality control is part of an integrated organizationwide program to assess and improve care.

ACTION PLAN[1,2,7]

The transition to organizationwide quality improvement will occur in stages and will take time. The stages will start with the top—leadership—and with acquiring a commitment to quality improvement. Next, quality improvement will filter down to management and will become more tangible through enumeration of priorities. Training for other employees follows, along with trial projects. Finally, quality

improvement activities reach all parts of the organization as does the cultural change of a new approach toward quality and a new cooperation.

Table 6 spells out this implementation process, along with estimated time frames.

A smooth, steady transition should not be expected. Although some staff will readily embrace quality improvement, others will be skeptical, based on the bad connotations of quality assurance. The cultural change that quality improvement aims toward is only earned over time by mounting evidence and experience showing quality improvement works. A strong leadership commitment and a sensible implementation plan will be necessary to weather the difficulties and earn the cultural change.

Each organization will need to tailor its implementation plan to its own needs and experiences, but the following are basic steps that should be considered.

1. Leadership Commitment

The transition will not take place if the leaders' commitment is not strong; the necessary investments in time, education, and so on will not occur, and the lack of belief will be communicated to the rest of the organization. Education in quality improvement and belief in its benefits are essential. (The Joint Commission's belief in the importance of education to quality improvement is shown in its choice of QA.1.1 as the one standard scored of QA.1 through QA.1.6 in 1992. QA.1.1 states, "The leaders undertake education concerning the approach and methods of continuous quality improvement.") A mission statement highlighting quality improvement will further solidify the commitment.

2. Acquire Expertise

The organization will have to make use of experts in quality improvement (whether as authors, consultants, or employees) to assure the program is ushered in efficiently and to assure the necessary skills are available for setting up a system to monitor, assess, and improve care and service.

3. Training Management in the Philosophies and Techniques of Quality Improvement

This training begins the process of exposing the staff from the top down to quality improvement. They, like the leaders, should know the basic beliefs of quality improvement and should be familiar with the methods, including basic statistical quality control.

4. Setting Priorities

The leaders, with others in the organization, should begin the search for the areas they need to improve. These areas for improvement should be based on data and should be placed in order of priority based on effect on patient care and resources necessary for improvement.

5. Further Training

All employees will need to know about quality improvement—its goals, the part they will play, the basics of statistical quality control. This training will prepare the organization for the next step.

6. Initial Projects

Some initial, possibly small-scale, projects should now start the process in motion. By keeping initial quality-improvement projects relatively simple, the organization can help produce some early successes, which should build faith in the process.

7. Initiate Projects Throughout the Organization

At this point, quality improvement projects should involve employees at all levels and in all parts of the organization. Employees should be actively involved in analyzing and

---

STAGES HOSPITALS UNDERGO TOWARD IMPLEMENTING QUALITY IMPROVEMENT

PHASE	TIME FRAME
Phase I	1 Year

- Leaders educate themselves by reading and taking courses on principles of CQI
- A mission statement that identifies CQI as an organizationwide commitment and goal is adopted by hospital leaders and promulgated throughout the organization

Phase II	1 Year

- Middle management is trained in the philosophy and methods of CQI
- Priorities are established for what the hospital will try to improve on (both opportunities to improve care and problems in care.) While staff from all levels of the organization are sometimes involved in discussing priorities, the actual selection of where time and money will be devoted is usually done by hospital leaders.

Phase III	2 Years

- Demo projects are initiated across departments
- Employees are trained in the methods and philosophy of CQI

Phase IV	2 Years

- Projects are initiated throughout the organization so that every employee is involved in the analysis of processes as they relate to outcomes
- Integration of efforts
- Cultural change

Source: Joint Commission: How to Achieve Quality and Accreditation in a Hospital Infection Control Program

Table 6

---

improving the processes in which they take part. Education for all staff, as necessary, should be ongoing.

8. Organizational Changes

The leaders and others involved in designing quality improvement should consider the structural changes that may be necessary to implement quality improvement. Such changes may involve giving a quality manager a central position in the organization. In particular, an effort should be made to assure quality improvement efforts throughout the organization are planned and coordinated.

9. Cultural Change

Finally, a cultural change should be achieved. This change will be seen in management that respects and supports all staff; in an awareness of how opportunities for improvement arise, how performance and processes are measured, and how they are improved; in an active, welcome involvement across the organization in quality improvement; and in increased cooperation and mutual respect.

EXAMPLES[7,8]

The extent to which quality improvement principles can be applied in health care organizations is being investigated and tested. As mentioned in Chapter One, under the National Demonstration Project, 21 health care organizations have been involved in exploring whether and how these industrial-based theories and practices can be applied. Experts in industrial quality control, who serve as consultants to the hospitals, report "that health care is just as riddled with operational quality defects as any other industry they have studied, and just as ripe for new forms of management and problem solving."[9]

Exactly how to apply quality improvement is still being investigated and debated. Most of the hospitals in the national project looked at individual system problems within their organizations and how to improve their processes. At Strong Memorial Hospital at the University of Rochester (NY) Medical Center, for example, staff uncovered two problems in their method of routing patients through the emergency department that caused unnecessarily long waiting times for some patients. After charting the flow of patients, they saw that "patients with simple problems were experiencing unnecessary delays, and the staff person in charge of patient care during the day was usually the most junior physician on the team." To resolve these problems, (1) more triage nurses were added for peak hours and cross training was begun for administrative and clerical staff, and (2) the senior faculty member took control of the emergency room team.[10]

While no health care organization has of yet completely integrated quality improvement into its organization or reached the final stage of cultural change, several hospitals

are beginning to make organizationwide changes (the step beyond simply addressing problems with a limited focus). West Paces Ferry Hospital in Atlanta, Georgia, has had a hospitalwide quality improvement program for three years. They just began involving their medical staff in the process. While the way in which hospitals adopt quality improvement might change, so far they have shown the same progression industries have gone through.

BEYOND THE PLAN

Having met the challenges of cost, involving leadership, involving staff, putting statistical quality control to work, and embarking on an action plan, organizations will still need to have carefully thought out the process by which care and service are monitored, assessed, and improved. Such a process is discussed in the next chapter.

REFERENCES

1. Crosby PB: Quality Without Tears. New York: McGraw-Hill, 1984.

2. Deming WE: Out of the Crisis. Cambridge, MA: Massachusetts Institute of Technology, 1986.

3. Berwick DM: Continuous improvement as an ideal in health care. N Engl J Med 320(1): 53-56.

4. Joint Commission on Accreditation of Healthcare Organizations: Quality Assurance in Managed Care Organizations. Chicago: Joint Commission, 1989.

5. Walton M: The Deming Management Method. New York: Dodd, Mead & Company, 1986.

6. Ishikawa K: What Is Total Quality Control? David J. Lu, trans. Englewood Cliffs, NJ: Prentice-Hall, Inc., 1985.

7. Joint Commission on Accreditation of Healthcare Organizations: Striving Toward Improvement. Oakbrook Terrace, IL: Joint Commission, 1990.

8. Joint Commission on Accreditation of Healthcare Organizations: How to Achieve Quality and Accreditation in a Hospital Infection Control Program. Oakbrook Terrace, IL: Joint Commission, 1990.

9. Berwick DM: Health services research and quality of care. Assignments for the 1990s. Med Care 27(8): 763-771, Aug 1989.

10. Lespare M: Is what's good for Ford Motor Company good for healthcare? Quality Letter, Sep 1987.

Chapter Five

ASSESSMENT AND IMPROVEMENT

Opportunities for improvement can be identified only through effective performance monitoring. Drawing upon existing QA principles, this requires the prudent selection and application of good performance measures or indicators.[1]

A process to assess and improve the quality of care and service is essential to quality improvement. Elsewhere in this book, the need to use statistical quality control methods in this process has been stated. The overall process is equally important.

In the last several years, the ten-step monitoring and evaluation process has been the Joint Commission's recommended means of assessing and improving the quality of care and service. Although the ten-step process isn't explicitly described in the Joint Commission's 1992 "Quality Assessment and Improvement" standards, many of its steps are still included. These steps will continue to be part of the standards through 1993; the 1994 standards will refer to ongoing monitoring, but will be less explicit about the way that monitoring is carried out.

As mentioned in Chapter One, quality improvement builds on the strengths of quality assurance, and monitoring and evaluation is clearly amenable to use in an organization-wide quality improvement program. Other assessment and improvement processes also are appropriate for quality improvement, and the Joint Commission encourages organizations to consider them. Readers should remember that the various methods have more in common than not. All involve focusing on particular areas in the organization, collecting data, evaluating performance of processes and outcomes, taking action for improvement, and assessing

improvement through further data collection. Joint Commission surveyors are knowledgeable in methods for quality improvement and will support organizations as they adapt their monitoring and evaluation activities for quality improvement or as they gradually move to another method to objectively assess and improve the quality of care and services.

MONITORING AND EVALUATION

The monitoring and evaluation process involves

- identifying the most important aspects of care and service an organization, a department, or a service provides;
- using measures—indicators—to systematically monitor these aspects of care and service in an ongoing way;
- evaluating the care and service, when predetermined levels or patterns, including trends, are reached, to identify opportunities to improve the quality of care and service; and
- taking actions to improve care and service or to solve problems, and evaluating the effectiveness of those actions.

Monitoring and evaluation is the process by which much quality-improvement activity can be carried out.

As discussed in Chapter One, quality assurance and monitoring and evaluation provide a solid point of departure for quality improvement. Before discussing how the monitoring and evaluation process can work in quality improvement, it will be useful to briefly revisit some of the modifications that will be necessary to the process, which were mentioned in Chapter One. The modifications will include

- emphasizing the leadership role in improving quality;
- expanding the scope of assessment and improvement activities beyond the strictly clinical to the interrelated governance, managerial, support, and clinical processes that affect patient outcomes;
- using other sources of feedback (in addition to ongoing monitoring) to trigger evaluation and improvement of care and service;
- organizing the assessment and improvement activities around the flow of patient care and service, with special attention to how the "customer and supplier" relationships between departments (as well as within departments) can be improved, rather than compartmentalizing activities within departments and services;
- focusing first on the processes of care and service rather than solely on the performance of individuals;
- emphasizing continuous improvement rather than only

solving identified problems; and

- maintaining improvement over time.

The description that follows shows how a revised monitoring and evaluation process addresses these issues to effectively contribute to continuous quality improvement.

Monitoring and evaluation comprises the following ten steps:

Step 1: Assign responsibility;

Step 2: Delineate scope of care and service;

Step 3: Identify important aspects of care and service;

Step 4: Identify indicators;

Step 5: Establish a means to trigger evaluation;

Step 6: Collect and organize data;

Step 7: Initiate evaluation;

Step 8: Take actions to improve care and service;

Step 9: Assess the effectiveness of actions and assure improvement is maintained; and

Step 10: Communicate results to relevant individuals and groups.

Figure 13 and Tables 7, 8, and 9 help elucidate this process.

THE MONITORING AND EVALUATION PROCESS

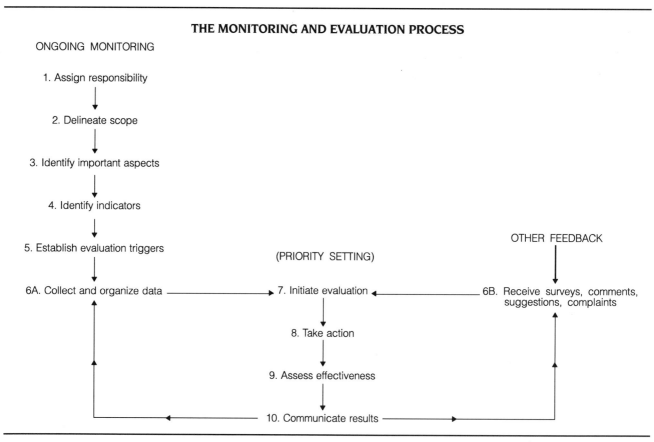

Figure 13
Graphic representation of the ten-step monitoring and evaluation process

OUTLINE OF THE MONITORING AND EVALUATION PROCESS

Step 1: **Assign responsibility**
- a. Identify organization leaders
- b. Design and foster approach to continuous improvement of quality
- c. Set priorities for assessment and improvement

Step 2: **Delineate scope of care and service**
- a. Identify key functions and/or identify the procedures, treatments, and other activities performed in the organization

Step 3: **Identify important aspects of care and service**
- a. Determine the key functions, treatments, processes, and other aspects of care and service that warrant ongoing monitoring
- b. Establish priorities among the important aspects of care and service chosen

Step 4: **Identify indicators**
- a. Identify teams to develop indicators for the important aspects of care and service
- b. Select indicators

Step 5: **Establish means to trigger evaluation**
- a. For each indicator, the team identifies how evaluation may be triggered
- b. Select the means to trigger evaluation

Step 6: **Collect and organize data**
- a. Each team identifies data sources and data-collection methods for the recommended indicators
- b. Design the final data-collection methodology, including those responsible for collection, organization, and determining whether evaluation is triggered
- c. Collect data
- d. Organize data to determine whether evaluation is required
- e. Collect data from other sources, including patient and staff surveys, comments, suggestions, and complaints

Step 7: **Initiate evaluation**
- a. Determine whether evaluation should be initiated
- b. Assess other feedback (eg, staff suggestions, patient-satisfaction survey results) that may contribute to priority setting for evaluation
- c. Set priorities for evaluation
- d. Teams undertake intensive evaluation

Step 8: **Take actions to improve care and service**
- a. Teams recommend and/or take actions

Step 9: **Assess the effectiveness of actions and assure improvement is maintained**
- a. Assess to determine whether care and service have improved
- b. If not, determine further action
- c. Repeat a) and b) until improvement is obtained and maintained
- d. Maintain monitoring
- e. Periodically reassess priorities for monitoring

Step 10: **Communicate results to relevant individuals and groups**
- a. Teams forward conclusions, actions, and results to leaders and to affected individuals, committees, department, and services
- b. Disseminate information as necessary
- c. Leaders and others receive and disseminate comments, reactions, and information from involved individuals and groups

Table 7

Figure 13 is a graphic depiction of the process as a whole. Table 7 presents the process in outline form and should help give readers an overview of monitoring and evaluation. Table 8 is a checklist to help organizations adequately design their monitoring and evaluation activities to benefit from the philosophy and methods of continuous quality improvement. Table 9 presents a brief look at the differences between the monitoring and evaluation process as currently practiced and the modified process explained here.

The monitoring and evaluation process includes both planning (Steps 1 through 5) and action (Steps 6 through 10). The following sections explain each step in more detail.

Step 1: Assign Responsibility

The organization leaders are responsible for (a) overseeing the design of a quality improvement system; (b) fostering an organizationwide commitment to quality improvement; (c) establishing quality-improvement responsibilities; and (d) setting strategic priorities for quality assessment and improvement.

Organization leaders. According to the 1992 "Quality Assessment and Improvement" standards, the organization's leaders include at least the following:

the leaders of the governing body; the chief executive officer and other senior managers; the elected and/or appointed leaders of the medical staff and the clinical departments, and other medical staff members in hospital administrative positions; and the nursing executive and other senior nursing leaders.[2]

Leadership involvement is key to achieving an organizationwide commitment to improving quality, to assuring that quality improvement is given high priority among the organization's activities, and to assuring that it includes those important processes that cross department/service lines.

Designing and fostering an approach to quality improvement. The organization leaders are responsible for overseeing the design of the organization's approach to improving quality and for ensuring that this approach is carried out. Designing the approach to continuously improving quality includes determining
- how the subjects of ongoing monitoring will be chosen;
- how other feedback about quality-related issues can be used to ascertain opportunities for improvement;
- how priorities for assessment and improvement will be set;
- how assessment and improvement methods will be used;

CHECKLIST FOR DESIGNING THE MONITORING AND EVALUATION PROCESS*

____ Have leaders been identified?

____ Has a structure been established for leaders to oversee quality-improvement activities?

Does the monitoring and evaluation process include

____ a delineation of the scope of care and service?

____ important aspects of care and service to be monitored on an ongoing basis?

____ a procedure to develop and approve indicators and evaluation triggers for each important aspect of care?

____ a data-collection methodology?

____ a procedure by which data are assessed to see whether evaluation is triggered?

____ a procedure by which other feedback (eg, patient and staff surveys) may trigger further evaluation?

____ a procedure by which actions are taken to improve care and service?

____ a procedure by which care and service are reassessed and improvement is maintained?

____ a procedure by which all affected individuals and groups receive results of monitoring and evaluation?

*This checklist pertains to designing, rather than performing, monitoring and evaluation. Conscientiously fulfilling all items on this checklist means the organization should have the basis for an effective monitoring and evaluation process for quality improvement.

Table 8

---

and
- how quality-related information will be disseminated throughout the organization.

The leaders must also determine how they will help all staff learn the methods of quality improvement and foster staff commitment to and involvement in the process.

Establishing responsibilities in the organization. Once the process for continuously improving quality has been designed, the leaders must establish who will be responsible for carrying out the process. No matter how and by whom the process is carried out, the leaders continue to oversee and, as appropriate, participate in the activities. Department/service directors are responsible for seeing that activities in their departments are encompassed by the monitoring and evaluation activities.

DISTINCTIONS BETWEEN THE MONITORING AND EVALUATION PROCESS AS CURRENTLY PRACTICED AND THE MONITORING AND EVALUATION PROCESS IN THE CONTEXT OF CONTINUOUS QUALITY IMPROVEMENT

Step 1: Assign responsibility

CURRENT:
Each department/service assigns responsibility for overseeing and carrying out monitoring and evaluation within the department.

QI:
The organization leaders oversee the design of and foster an approach to continuously improving quality that includes both intradepartmental and interdepartmental activities.

Step 2: Delineate scope of care and service

CURRENT:
Each department/service delineates its separate scope of care.

QI:
The organization, as a whole or by department/service, delineates its scope of care and service.

Step 3: Identify important aspects of care and service

CURRENT:
Each department/service identifies its high-volume, high-risk, and problem-prone aspects of care.

QI:
The organization, as a whole or by department/service, identifies high-priority important functions, processes, treatments, activities, and so forth, to be monitored.

Step 4: Identify indicators

CURRENT:
Each department/service identifies indicators to correspond to the important aspects of care.

QI:
Teams of experts, inter- or intradepartmental, identify indicators for the important aspects of care and service. Indicators pertaining to structures of care are less emphasized.

Step 5: Establish a means to trigger evaluation

CURRENT:
Each department/service establishes the level or pattern in data for each indicator that would trigger intensive evaluation.

QI:
Teams of experts establish the level or pattern in data for each indicator that will trigger intensive evaluation. Statistical methods are emphasized, as is the fact that performance levels of process and outcomes are not the only way evaluation is triggered.

Step 6: Collect and organize data

CURRENT:
The department/service or organization establishes a data-collection methodology.

QI:
The data-collection methodology often includes a means by which feedback from sources other than ongoing monitoring is used to indicate areas for evaluation and improvement.

Step 7: Initiate evaluation

CURRENT:
Care is intensively evaluated only when the threshold for a given indicator is reached.

QI:
When the level or pattern in the data triggers evaluation, and also when other feedback (eg, patient reports, staff reports) identifies other opportunities for improvement, leaders set priorities for evaluation and establish teams, which evaluate the patient care or service function in question.

Step 8: Take actions to improve care and service

CURRENT:
Those with authority within or outside the department/service take action, based on recommendations of those who evaluate the care.

QI:
Greater emphasis is placed on focusing actions on processes, especially the "hand offs" between departments/services.

Step 9: Assess the effectiveness of actions and assure improvement is maintained

CURRENT:
Continued monitoring determines whether actions are effective.

QI:
A greater emphasis is placed on assuring that improvement is sustained over time through changes in processes, as well as continued data collection.

Step 10: Communicate results to affected individuals and groups

CURRENT:
Departments/services and functions report results to the quality assurance program, which disseminates the findings, as necessary.

QI:
Findings of those performing monitoring and evaluation are forwarded to the leaders and to affected individuals and groups. Leaders also disseminate information, as necessary.

Table 9

Setting priorities. Among the leaders' most important responsibilities is overseeing the setting of priorities for assessment and improvement. Priority setting is based on review of findings from ongoing monitoring as well as other feedback that may indicate an opportunity to improve the quality of care and service. After consideration of the effect of each aspect of care and service on patients, and of organization resources, the priorities should be set for evaluation and, as appropriate, improvement.

Step 2: Delineate Scope of Care and Service

All care and service the organization provides patients should be considered when setting priorities for ongoing monitoring.

Identifying important functions. One method of delineating the scope of care and service is to identify the organization's important governance, managerial, clinical, and support functions. All departments and services should contribute to this delineation of important functions.

Important functions are those functions that have the greatest effect on the quality of care the patient ultimately receives, including clinical, support, managerial, and governance activities. Such important functions could include, among others,

- leadership;
- human resources management;
- information management;
- environmental management;
- quality assessment and improvement;
- patient rights;
- admission to setting or service;
- patient evaluation;
- nutritional care;
- operative and other invasive procedures;
- nonoperative treatment selection and administration;
- patient and family education; and
- transfer, discharge, and aftercare.

If the organization chooses this method of delineating its scope of care and service, the focus of quality improvement will be on understanding and improving the processes that compose these important functions.

(A focus on important functions is not required by the Joint Commission. By 1994, however, standards in the Accreditation Manual for Hospitals will be progressively organized around important functions, which should be among those the hospital addresses in its quality improvement activities.)

Identifying activities. Another method of delineating scope of care and service is to compile an inventory of the activities performed in the organization. Such an inventory can be based on a review of the

- types of patients served;
- range of conditions and diagnoses treated;
- range of activities involved in serving patients (including activities other than direct patient care);
- types of staff carrying out these activities;
- sites where care and service are provided; and
- times when care and service are provided.

If the organization uses this method to delineate scope of care and service, quality improvement focuses on understanding and improving the functions and processes involved in the various activities.

Step 3: Identify Important Aspects of Care and Service

In this step, the organization chooses the subjects for ongoing monitoring and determines their priorities.

Selecting the aspects of care and service that will be monitored. Using the scope of care and service as a basis, the organization selects those aspects of care and service important enough to warrant ongoing monitoring. These aspects of care may be important functions, procedures, treatments, processes, or other activities that affect patient care.

The choice of important aspects of care or service should be made by those who are experts in the areas under consideration, and the organization leaders should concur with their choice. The aspects of care chosen should be those believed most important to the quality of patient care and service. Organization resources and the importance to patients are factors to consider in determining what can and should be monitored.

The following are examples of some possible important aspects of care and service (these example all pertain to medication use):

- Medication ordering;
- Medication preparation and dispensing;
- Medication administration;
- Monitoring of medication effects;
- Emergency drug distribution;
- Screening and monitoring for drug sensitivities;
- IV admixture preparation;
- Drawing peak and trough serum drug levels; and
- Counseling patients.

Establishing priorities. Leaders and those expert in the aspects of care should set priorities for monitoring. Again, organization resources and importance to patient care will be factors to consider.

Step 4: Identify Indicators[3]

This step involves selecting the performance measures for the important aspects of care and service. The following paragraphs offer a brief summary of how indicators are developed and used. A complete treatment of this subject can be found in Primer on Indicator Development and Application, available from the Joint Commission.

What are indicators? An indicator is a quantitative measure that can be used to assess and improve the performance of important governance, management, clinical, and support functions that affect patient outcomes. An indicator is not a direct measure of quality. Rather, it is a tool that can be used to assess performance and that can direct attention to potential performance issues that may require more intense review within an organization.

For specified patient care activities, indicators may direct attention to one or more of a range of patient care components, including accessibility, appropriateness, continuity of care, effectiveness, efficacy, efficiency, patient perspective issues, safety of the care environment, and timeliness.

Process and outcome indicators. Indicators may assess an outcome or a process of care. An outcome indicator assesses what happens or does not happen following a process (for example, the patient's condition after a patient care function is performed or not performed). An example of an outcome indicator is "patients who fail to emerge from general anesthesia within one hour of termination of anesthesia." Patient mortality or survival (that is, what happens to the patient) with respect to care functions performed or not performed are additional examples of outcome indicators.

A process indicator assesses an important and discrete activity that is carried out, either to directly care for the patient (for example, patient assessment) or to support patient care (for example, determining that practitioners perform competently). The best of such indicators identify processes that are linked to patient outcomes, meaning that a scientific basis exists for believing that the process, when provided effectively, increases the probability of a desired outcome. An example of a process indicator is "female patients with American Joint Committee on Cancer pathological Stage II lymph node positive primary invasive breast cancer not treated with systemic adjuvant therapy." The use of systemic or radiation adjuvant therapy as part of the female breast cancer patient management process has been shown to improve overall long-term survival, or outcome (that is, five-year survival rates), for this group of patients. The provision of adjuvant therapy is a discrete process of care; its omission is expected to have an adverse effect on long-term survival rates and suggests that an opportunity for improvement in the quality of care exists.

An outcome or a process indicator may be used to assess an event that is either desirable or undesirable. An example of an outcome indicator that assesses a desirable event is "survival of patients at 1, 3, and 5 years with primary cancer of the lung, colon/rectum, or female breast by stage and histologic type." An example of an outcome indicator that assesses an undesirable event is "patients who die during or within 48 hours following the administration of anesthesia."

Rate-based and sentinel event indicators. An indicator may express information (1) as the rate at which events occur within a defined universe over time, or (2) to draw attention to individual occurrences of events.

When the rate format is used to describe indicator information, the indicator is called a *rate-based indicator*. The numerator of the rate is the number of patients for whom the indicator event occurs; the denominator is the number of patients who have the condition or procedure the indicator is assessing. In virtually all cases, a rate-based indicator assesses an event for which a certain proportion of the events that occur are expected (see the next section on how evaluation is triggered).

An example of a rate-based indicator is "patients receiving primary cesarean section for failure to progress." In this case, the numerator would be the number of events this indicator identifies; the denominator would be the number of patients who receive a primary cesarean section. Failure to progress is an appropriate reason for performing primary cesarean sections in a proportion of patients receiving primary cesarean sections. Individual case review, however, should be initiated when a predetermined threshold has been crossed or a pattern (for example, a trend) in the data has been identified.

Unlike rate-based indicators, *sentinel-event indicators* identify specific "serious" events that require case-by-case analysis every time they occur. An example of a sentinel-event indicator is "patients who die as a result of blood transfusions." This serious outcome of care is almost always unacceptable and should almost never occur, given the current state of the art.

The event is sufficiently serious that thorough investigation of the clinical decisions and support service processes linked to the event must take place for each occurrence.

Table 10 offers some examples of indicators that could be used in monitoring and evaluation for quality improvement. These are the Joint Commission's anesthesia, obstetrics, cardiology, oncology, and trauma indicators, developed as part of the Agenda for Change initiatives.

Teams to identify indicators. To ensure that the most accurate and productive indicators are used, those staff who are knowledgeable about (and, usually, involved in) the particular aspects of care or service should work together. These teams of knowledgeable individuals may be interdepartmental or intradepartmental; each may address one or more aspects of care or service. Input from someone knowledgeable in the techniques of statistical quality control can be valuable.

A team should try to identify the processes that make up the important aspect of care or service to determine what measures would be most useful in monitoring it. In doing so, the team should consult authoritative sources, including health care literature, quality assurance/improvement literature, professional standards, and their own and other staff's experiences.

Choosing the best teams for indicator development will help all staff know the indicators are useful and accurate, resulting in increased faith and cooperation in quality improvement.

The Primer on Indicator Development and Application presents a detailed two-phase developmental process for indicators.[3] The first phase involves a subset of the full group of experts, including the methodology experts and selected content experts. Because organizations and their needs are unique, the specific identity of these experts may vary. In certain instances, the organization may choose to meet these needs through external consultation. The second phase is characterized by expansion of the subgroup to include additional content experts. The addition of other content experts provides for broadened perspectives on important issues and permits early involvement and education of a larger number of professionals who will be using the indicators. In small organizations, it may be practical to consolidate the two work phases.

Developing indicators. The first phase involves seven tasks:
1. Selection of the group leader or chairperson;
2. Development of the charge to the full group;
3. Preliminary definition of the scope of care to be monitored;
4. Preliminary identification of important aspects of care for which indicators should be developed;
5. Development of a preliminary set of indicators;
6. Development of indicator information sets (indicator statement, definition of terms, identification of indicator type, rationale for use of the indicator, description of the indicator population, indicator data-collection logic, and underlying factors that may explain variations in indicator data); and
7. Selection of additional content experts to serve in the full group.

The second phase has five major tasks:
1. Review and revision of the scope of care and important aspects of care;
2. Review of group composition;
3. Review, revision (including additions and deletions), and finalization of the set of indicators;
4. Definition of data elements for each indicator; and
5. Identification of underlying factors that may explain variation in performance.

Step 5: Establish a Means to Trigger Evaluation[3]

In this step, the organization establishes, for each indicator, a mechanism to determine when further evaluation must be triggered. In other words, the means to trigger evaluation should answer the question, "Based on these data, must we launch an intensive evaluation of this aspect of care?" (Action to improve care and service may of course be taken even when not triggered by a specified means.)

Single events and rates. By definition, a sentinel-event indicator identifies an event that triggers intensive evaluation each time the event it occurs. Triggers for rate-based indicators are less self-evident. One way to determine the rate that triggers evaluation is by expert consensus. This approach involves using sources such as clinical and quality assurance literature, external data bases, and/or in-house clinical judgment to determine expected rates for the monitored activity. Another method is for individual organizations to define their own objectives for performance relating to a given indicator. Yet another approach involves using a derived range around a statistical mean (calculated from data collected and adjusted, when necessary, for case mix). This approach involves use of statistics and requires a central data base that allows progressive accumulation of data and calculation of the statistical mean and a range around that mean (upper and lower control limits). A specified variation from the mean would trigger further evaluation.

JOINT COMMISSION ANESTHESIA, OBSTETRICS, CARDIOVASCULAR, ONCOLOGY, AND TRAUMA INDICATORS

This appendix contains the Joint Commission's anesthesia, obstetrics, cardiovascular, oncology, and trauma indicators. These indicators were developed over a three-and-a-half-year period and submitted to rigorous field testing. The Board of Commissioners has recommended that all hospitals providing such services consider using these indicators in their monitoring and evaluation programs.

Scoring guidelines for QA.3.1.2 through QA.3.1.2.1.1.3 in the "Quality Assessment and Improvement" chapter of this Manual (which requires hospitals to identify indicators for monitoring the quality of important aspects of care) stipulate that hospitals *at least consider* implementing any set(s) of indicators that the Joint Commission recommends. As of July 1, 1990, surveyors began using these scoring guidelines to evaluate compliance with the quality assessment and improvement standards that address monitoring and evaluation of the quality of care in hospitals.

See the "Quality Assessment and Improvement" chapter of the 1992 Accreditation Manual for Hospitals, Volume II for complete scoring guidelines to QA.3.1 through QA.3.1.7.2 concerning monitoring and evaluation activities.

ANESTHESIA CARE

AN-1 Patients developing a CNS complication occurring during or within two post-procedure days of procedures involving anesthesia administration, subcategorized by ASA-PS class, patient age, and CNS verses non-CNS related procedures.

AN-2 Patients developing a peripheral neurologic deficit during or within two post-procedure days of procedures involving anesthesia administration.

AN-3 Patients developing an acute myocardial infarction during or within two post-procedure days of procedures involving anesthesia administration, subcategorized by ASA-PS class, patient age, and cardiac versus non-cardiac procedures.

AN-4 Patients with a cardiac arrest during or within one post-procedure day of procedures involving anesthesia administration, excluding patients with required intraoperative cardiac arrest, subcategorized by ASA-PS class, patient age, and cardiac versus non-cardiac procedures.

AN-5 Patients with unplanned respiratory arrest during or within one post-procedure day of procedures involving anesthesia administration.

AN-6 Death of patients during or within two post-procedure days of procedures involving anesthesia administration, subcategorized by ASA-PS class and patient age.

AN-7 Unplanned admission of patients to the hospital within one post-procedure day following outpatient procedures involving anesthesia administration.

AN-8 Unplanned admission of patients to an intensive care unit within one post-procedure day of procedures involving anesthesia administration and with ICU stay greater than one day.

ADDITIONAL ANESTHESIA INDICATORS
(Not Retained for Beta Testing)

AN-A Patients with a discharge diagnosis of fulminant pulmonary edema developed during procedures involving anesthesia administration or within one post-procedure day of its conclusion.

AN-B Patients diagnosed with an aspiration pneumonitis occurring during procedures involving anesthesia administration or within two post-procedure days of its conclusion.

AN-C Patients developing a postural headache within four post-procedure days following procedures involving spinal or epidural anesthesia administration.

AN-D Patients experiencing a dental injury during procedures involving anesthesia care.

AN-E Patients experiencing an ocular injury during procedures involving anesthesia care.

OBSTETRICAL INDICATORS

OB-1 Patients with primary cesarean section for failure to progress.

OB-2 Patients with attempted vaginal birth after cesarean section (VBAC), subcategorized by success or failure.

OB-3 Patients with excessive maternal blood loss defined by either post-delivery red blood cell transfusion *or* a low post-delivery hematocrit or hemoglobin (Hct 22%, Hgb < 7 gms) *or* a significant pre- to post-delivery decrease in hematocrit (decrease 11%) or hemoglobin (decrease 3.5 gms) excluding patients with abruptio placentae or placenta previa.

OB-4 Patients with a diagnosis of eclampsia.

OB-5 The delivery of infants weighing less than 2500 grams, following either induction of labor or repeat cesarean section without medical indications.*

* *A list of the specific diagnoses and appropriate ICD-9-CM diagnostic codes for medical indications for induction of labor and repeat cesareans, for major congenital anomalies, and for significant birth trauma will be provided with the data element specifications for the obstetrics indicators.*

Continued on page 48

Table 10

JOINT COMMISSION ANESTHESIA, OBSTETRICS, CARDIOVASCULAR, ONCOLOGY, AND TRAUMA INDICATORS

OBSTETRICAL INDICATORS (cont.)

OB-6 Term infants admitted to an NICU within one day of delivery and with NICU stay greater than one day excluding admissions for major congenital anomalies.*

OB-7 Neonates with an Apgar score of three (3) or less at five (5) minutes and a birthweight greater than 1500 grams.

OB-8 Neonates with a discharge diagnosis of significant birth trauma.*

OB-9 Term infants with a diagnosis of hypoxic encephalopathy or clinically apparent seizure prior to discharge from the hospital of birth, excluding newborns with a diagnosis of fetal alcohol syndrome, and other drug reactions and withdrawal syndromes.

OB-10 Deaths of infants weighing 500 grams or more subcategorized by intrahospital neonatal deaths, total stillborns and intrapartum stillborns.

ADDITIONAL OBSTETRICAL INDICATORS
(Not Retained for Beta Testing)

OB-A Intrahospital neonatal deaths of infants with a birthweight of 750-999 grams born in a hospital with an NICU.

OB-B Maternal readmissions within 14 days of delivery.

OB-C Intrahospital maternal deaths occurring within 42 days postpartum.

OB-D Infants weighing less than 1800 grams delivered in a hospital without an NICU.

OB-E Neonates transferred from a non-NICU hospital to a NICU hospital.

CARDIOVASCULAR INDICATORS

Cardiovascular Patient Population: The cardiovascular indicators draw from four populations described below: coronary artery bypass grafts (CABG), percutaneous transluminal coronary angioplasty (PTCA), acute myocardial infarction (MI), and congestive heart failure (CHF).

CABG Patient Population: Patients undergoing CABG excluding those with other cardiac or peripheral vascular surgical procedures performed at the time of the CABG (eg, valve replacement).

CV-1 INDICATOR FOCUS: Intrahospital mortality as a means of assessing multiple aspects of CABG care.
Indicator (Numerator): Intrahospital mortality of patients undergoing isolated CABG procedures, subcategorized by initial

and subsequent CABG procedures, emergent or nonemergent clinical status and by postoperative day and intrahospital location of death.

CV-2 INDICATOR FOCUS: Extended postoperative stay as a means of assessing multiple aspects of CABG care.
Indicator (Numerator): Patients with prolonged postoperative stay for isolated CABG procedures subcategorized by initial or subsequent CABG procedures, emergent or nonemergent procedures and by the use or nonuse of a circulatory support device.

PTCA Patient Population: Patients for whom a PTCA procedure is initiated, regardless of whether or not a lesion is crossed or dilated.

CV-3 INDICATOR FOCUS: Intrahospital mortality as a means of assessing multiple aspects of PTCA care.
Indicator (Numerator): Intrahospital mortality of patients following PTCA subcategorized by emergent or nonemergent clinical status and by postprocedure day and intrahospital location of death.

CV-4 INDICATOR FOCUS: Specific clinical events as a means of assessing multiple aspects of PTCA care.
Indicator (Numerator): Patients undergoing nonemergent PTCA with subsequent occurrence of either an acute MI or CABG procedure within the same hospitalization.

CV-5 INDICATOR FOCUS: Effectiveness of PTCA.
Indicator (Numerator): Patients undergoing attempted or completed PTCA during which any lesion attempted is not dilated.

MI Patient Population: Patients with a principal diagnosis of acute MI either upon hospital discharge, emergency department (ED) transfer to another acute care facility, or death in the ED, and patients who are admitted for an acute MI or to rule out an acute MI.

CV-6 INDICATOR FOCUS: Intrahospital mortality as a means of assessing multiple aspects of acute MI care.
Indicator (Numerator): Intrahospital mortality of patients with principal discharge diagnosis of acute MI subcategorized by history of previous infarction, age, and intrahospital location of death.

A list of the specific diagnoses and appropriate ICD-9-CM diagnostic codes for medical indications for induction of labor and repeat cesareans, for major congenital anomalies, and for significant birth trauma will be provided with the data element specifications for the obstetrics indicators.

Continued on page 49

Table 10

JOINT COMMISSION ANESTHESIA, OBSTETRICS, CARDIOVASCULAR, ONCOLOGY, AND TRAUMA INDICATORS

CARDIOVASCULAR INDICATORS (cont.)

CV-7 INDICATOR FOCUS: Diagnostic accuracy and resource utilization.
Indicator (Numerator): Patients admitted for acute MI, to rule out acute MI, or for unstable angina who have a discharge diagnosis of acute MI subcategorized by admission to an intensive care unit, a monitored bed, or an unmonitored bed.

CHF Patient Population: Patients with a discharge diagnosis of CHF with or without specific etiologies.

CV-8 INDICATOR FOCUS: Diagnostic accuracy.
Indicator (Numerator): Patients with discharge diagnosis of CHF with documented etiology and chest x-ray substantiation of CHF.

CV-9 INDICATOR FOCUS: Monitoring patient's response to therapy.
Indicator (Numerator): Patients with a principal discharge diagnosis of CHF and with at least two determinations of patient weight and of serum sodium, potassium, blood urea nitrogen, and creatinine levels.

ADDITIONAL CARDIOVASCULAR INDICATORS
(Not Retained for Beta Testing)

CV-A INDICATOR FOCUS: Specific complication of CABG as a means of assessing the management of CABG patients.
Indicator (Numerator): Patients undergoing isolated CABG procedures returning to the operating room for treatment of postoperative thoracic bleeding subcategorized by presence or absence of thrombolytic therapy received within 48 hours prior to CABG.

CV-B INDICATOR FOCUS: Specific complication of CABG as a means of assessing multiple aspects of CABG care.
Indicator (Numerator): Intra- or postoperative cerebrovascular accident in patients undergoing isolated CABG procedure.

CV-C INDICATOR FOCUS: Effectiveness of PTCA.
Indicator (Numerator): Patients with repeat PTCA of the same lesion occurring within 72 hours of the most recent PTCA subcategorized by emergent and nonemergent status of original PTCA.

CV-D INDICATOR FOCUS: Specific complication of PTCA as a means of assessing multiple aspects of PTCA care.
Indicator (Numerator): Patients with post-PTCA complications at femoral or brachial artery insertion site subcategorized by thrombolytic therapy within 48 hours prior to PTCA.

CV-E INDICATOR FOCUS: Management of thrombolytic therapy in patients with acute MI.
Indicator (Numerator): Hemorrhagic complications in patients receiving thrombolytic therapy for acute MI

subcategorized by complications occurring to patients prior to discharge from the institution initiating therapy and posttransfer complications occurring to patients who received therapy prior to transfer.

ONCOLOGY INDICATORS

Oncology Patient Population: Inpatients admitted for initial diagnosis and/or treatment of primary lung, colon, rectal, or female breast cancer.

ON-1 INDICATOR FOCUS: Availability of data for diagnosis and staging.
Indicator (Numerator): Surgical pathology consultation reports (pathology reports) containing histologic type, tumor size, status of margins, appropriate lymph node examination, assessment of invasion or extension as indicated, and AJCC/pTN classification for patients with resection for primary cancer of the lung, colon/rectum, or female breast.

ON-2 INDICATOR FOCUS: Use of staging by managing physicians.
Indicator (Numerator): Patients undergoing treatment for primary cancer of the lung, colon/rectum, or female breast with AJCC stage of tumor designated by a managing physician.

ON-3 INDICATOR FOCUS: Effectiveness of cancer treatment.
Indicator (Numerator): Survival of patients with primary cancer of the lung, colon/rectum, or female breast by stage and histologic type.*

ON-4 INDICATOR FOCUS: Use of tests critical to diagnosis, prognosis and clinical management.
Indicator (Numerator): Female patients with invasive primary breast cancer undergoing initial biopsy or resection of a tumor larger than one centimeter in greatest dimension who have presence of estrogen receptor diagnostic analysis results in medical record.

ON-5 INDICATOR FOCUS: Use of multimodal therapy in treatment and follow-up.
Indicator (Numerator): Female patients with AJCC Stage II pathologic lymph node positive primary invasive breast cancer treated with systemic adjuvant therapy.

ON-6 INDICATOR FOCUS: Effectiveness of preoperative diagnosis and staging.
Indicator (Numerator): Patients with non-small-cell primary lung cancer undergoing thoracotomy with complete surgical resection of tumor.

*Efficient mechanisms to obtain postdischarge data will be explored only with a subset of beta test hospitals. Ability to obtain these data during beta testing is not a requirement for participation.

Continued on page 50

Table 10

JOINT COMMISSION ANESTHESIA, OBSTETRICS, CARDIOVASCULAR, ONCOLOGY, AND TRAUMA INDICATORS

ONCOLOGY INDICATORS (cont.)

ON-7 INDICATOR FOCUS: Specific clinical events as a means of assessing multiple aspects of surgical care for lung cancers.
Indicator (Numerator): Patients undergoing pulmonary resection for primary lung cancer with postoperative complication of empyema, broncho-pleural fistula, reoperation for postoperative bleeding, mechanical ventilation greater than five days postoperatively, or intrahospital death.

ON-8 INDICATOR FOCUS: Comprehensiveness of diagnostic workup.
Indicator (Numerator): Patients with resections of primary colorectal cancer whose preoperative evaluation by a managing physician includes examination of the entire colon, liver function tests, chest x-ray, and carcinoembryonic antigen levels.

ON-9 INDICATOR FOCUS: Documentation of staging, prognosis, and surgical treatment.
Indicator (Numerator): Patients with resection of primary colorectal cancer whose operative reports include location of primary tumor, local extent of disease, extent of resection, and assessment of residual abdominal disease.

ON-10 INDICATOR FOCUS: Use of treatment approaches which impact on quality of life.
Indicator (Numerator): Patients with primary rectal cancer undergoing abdominoperineal resections with 6 cm or more of free distal surgical margin present on specimen, as documented in surgical pathology gross description.

ON-11 INDICATOR FOCUS: Interdisciplinary treatment and follow-up.
Indicator (Numerator): Patients with AJCC Stage II or III primary rectal cancer with documentation of referral to or treatment by a radiation or medical oncologist.

ADDITIONAL ONCOLOGY INDICATORS
(Not Retained for Beta Testing)

ON-A INDICATOR FOCUS: Availability of specific data needed for diagnosis.
Indicator (Numerator): Presence of a written pathology report in the medical record of the treating institution documenting the pathologic diagnosis of patients receiving initial treatment for primary lung, colorectal, or female breast cancer.

ON-B INDICATOR FOCUS: Symptomatic and/or palliative care.
Indicator (Numerator): Systematic initial assessment of pain for all patients hospitalized due to metastatic lung, colorectal, or female breast cancer with pain.

ON-C INDICATOR FOCUS: Use of clinical staging.
Indicator (Numerator): Presence of documented AJCC clinical staging in the medical record prior to the first course of therapy for female patients with primary breast cancer.

ON-D INDICATOR FOCUS: Use of multimodal therapy in treatment and follow-up.
Indicator (Numerator): Treatment of female patients with primary invasive AJCC clinical Stage I or II breast cancer by excisional biopsy, segmental mastectomy, or quadrantectomy without radiation therapy.

ON-E INDICATOR FOCUS: Use of psychosocial support for patient follow-up.
Indicator (Numerator): Referral to support or rehabilitation groups or provision of psychosocial support for female patients with primary breast cancer.

ON-F INDICATOR FOCUS: Patient education.
Indicator (Numerator): Patients undergoing resection for primary colorectal cancer with enterostomy present at discharge who demonstrate understanding of enterostomy care and management instructions.

TRAUMA INDICATORS

Trauma Patient Population: Patients with ICD-9-CM diagnostic code of 800 through 959.9 who either are admitted to the hospital, die in the emergency department (ED), or are transferred from the hospital or the ED to another acute care facility, excluding patients with the following isolated injuries: burns; hip fractures in the elderly; specified fractures of the face, hand, and foot; and specified eye wounds.

TR-1 INDICATOR FOCUS: Efficiency of emergency medical services (EMS).
Indicator (Numerator): Trauma patients with prehospital EMS scene time greater than 20 minutes.

TR-2 INDICATOR FOCUS: Ongoing monitoring of trauma patients.
Indicator (Numerator): Trauma patients with blood pressure, pulse, respiration, and Glasgow Coma Scale (GCS) documented in the ED record on arrival and hourly until inpatient admission to operating room or intensive care unit, death, or transfer to another care facility (hourly GCS needed only if altered state of consciousness).

TR-3 INDICATOR FOCUS: Airway management of comatose trauma patients.
Indicator (Numerator): Comatose patients discharged from the ED prior to the establishment of a mechanical airway.

Continued on page 51

Table 10

JOINT COMMISSION ANESTHESIA, OBSTETRICS, CARDIOVASCULAR, ONCOLOGY, AND TRAUMA INDICATORS

TRAUMA INDICATORES (cont.)

TR-4 INDICATOR FOCUS: Timeliness of diagnostic testing.
Indicator (Numerator): Trauma patients with diagnosis of intracranial injury and altered state of consciousness upon ED arrival receiving initial head computerized tomography scan greater than two hours after ED arrival.

TR-5 INDICATOR FOCUS: Timeliness of surgical intervention for adult head injury.
Indicator (Numerator): Trauma patients with diagnosis of extradural or subdural brain hemorrhage undergoing craniotomy greater than four hours after ED arrival (excluding intracranial pressure monitoring) subcategorized by pediatric or adult patients.

TR-6 INDICATOR FOCUS: Timeliness of surgical intervention for orthopedic injuries.
Indicator (Numerator): Trauma patients with open fractures of the long bones as a result of blunt trauma receiving initial surgical treatment greater than eight hours after ED arrival.

TR-7 INDICATOR FOCUS: Timeliness of surgical intervention for abdominal injuries.
Indicator (Numerator): Trauma patients with diagnosis of laceration of the liver or spleen, requiring surgery, undergoing laparotomy greater than two hours after ED arrival, subcategorized by pediatric or adult patients.

TR-8 INDICATOR FOCUS: Surgical decision making for abdominal gunshot wounds versus stab wounds.
Indicator (Numerator): Trauma patients undergoing laparotomy for wounds penetrating the abdominal wall subcategorized by gunshot versus stab wounds.

TR-9 INDICATOR FOCUS: Timeliness of patient transfers.
Indicator (Numerator): Trauma patients transferred from initial receiving hospital to another acute care facility within six hours from ED arrival to ED departure.

TR-10 INDICATOR FOCUS: Surgical decision making for orthopedic injuries.
Indicator (Numerator): Adult trauma patients with femoral diaphyseal fractures treated by a nonfixation technique.

TR-11 INDICATOR FOCUS: Clinical decision making for potentially preventable deaths.
Indicator (Numerator): Intrahospital mortality of trauma patients—with one or more of the following conditions—who did not undergo a procedure for the condition: tension pneumothorax, hemoperitoneum, hemothoraces, ruptured aorta, pericardial tamponade, and epidural or subdural hemorrhage.

TR-12 INDICATOR FOCUS: Systems necessary for obtaining autopsies for trauma victims.
Indicator (Numerator): Trauma patients who expired within 48 hours of ED arrival for whom an autopsy was performed.

ADDITIONAL TRAUMA INDICATORS
(Not Retained for Beta Testing)

TR-A INDICATOR FOCUS: Communication between EMS and ED.
Indicator (Numerator): Copy of ambulance run report(s) not present with ED medical record for trauma patients transported by prehospital EMS personnel.

TR-B INDICATOR FOCUS: Trauma patient assessments in the emergency department.
Indicator (Numerator): Trauma patients admitted through the ED with inpatient discharge diagnosis of cervical spine injury not indicated in admission diagnosis.

TR-C INDICATOR FOCUS: Emergency department decision making.
Indicator (Numerator): Death of trauma patients with discharge diagnosis of closed pelvic fracture who receive transfusions of greater than six units of blood.

TR-D INDICATOR FOCUS: Clinical decision making for surgical intervention.
Indicator (Numerator): Trauma patients receiving initial abdominal, thoracic, vascular, or cranial surgery (excluding orthopedic, plastic, and hand surgery) more than 24 hours after ED arrival.

TR-E INDICATOR FOCUS: Use of blood products.
Indicator (Numerator): Transfusion of platelets and/or fresh frozen plasma within 24 hours of ED arrival in adult trauma patients receiving less than eight units of packed red blood cells or whole blood.

TR-F INDICATOR FOCUS: Effectiveness of surgical intervention.
Indicator (Numerator): Return of trauma patients to the operating room within 48 hours of completion of initial surgery.

TR-G INDICATOR FOCUS: Clinical decision making for femoral shaft fractures.
Indicator (Numerator): Trauma patients with femoral diaphyseal fractures that are not associated with other injuries who do not receive physical therapy or rehabilitation therapy.

Note: The final wording of each indicator in this appendix may be subject to revision based on the results of further testing.

Table 10

Patterns/trends. Patterns, including trends, in the data also may be used to trigger evaluation. Observing trends means observing data collected over time. These data may not show a trend, may show performance moving in a desirable direction, or may show performance moving in an undesirable direction. In case of the latter, evaluation may be initiated in an attempt to explain and change the trend.

Staff may also discern other patterns that suggest the need for intensive evaluation. For example, a certain indicator event may be found to occur more often during a certain shift or shifts. Although the aggregate performance rate may be seen as satisfactory, such a pattern could signal a possible opportunity for improvement.

(In addition, as discussed under steps 6 and 7, other feedback from staff, patients, or other sources may trigger intensive evaluation.)

All indicators should have some means to trigger evaluation. Each team charged with developing indicators may also establish this means.

Step 6: *Collect and Organize Data*

For each indicator, data are collected and organized so those responsible can determine when further evaluation is required.

Identifying data sources. The individual, group, or teams that develop indicators are in the best position to identify sources for data pertaining to each indicator. This information helps guide a decision about which indicators will be most productive and what data-collection methodology is appropriate. The source of data will vary depending on the indicator, but the following are some common places quality-related data can be found:

- Patients' records;
- Laboratory reports;
- Incident reports;
- Medication sheets;
- Department logs;
- Autopsy reports;
- Infection control reports;
- Direct observation and measurement; and
- Utilization review findings.

Each organization should work to assure that these data sources contain the most complete and accurate data possible. For example, patient complications should be well defined and consistently recorded.

Data-collection methodology. A data-collection methodology should be chosen and established. Because data collection that follows the flow of patient care often crosses departmental lines and involves the entire organization, cross-departmental teams or leaders often oversee design of the data-collection methods. Expertise in statistical quality control will be helpful. To minimize the investment of organization resources, the most efficient data-collection process should be established—one that takes into account data-collection already being carried out in the organization.

Designing and establishing this methodology entail answering several related questions:
- Who will collect data?
- Will collection be concurrent, retrospective, or both?
- Will sampling be appropriate?
- Is data collection amenable to computer support?
- How often will data be organized and assessed to note when evaluation is necessary?
- Who will organize data?
- How will data be displayed?
- Who will initiate evaluation?

To decide who will collect data and how they will be collected, the responsible individuals should look at existing activities that involve data collection, including utilization review, medical record abstracting, and so on. Ideally, data collection for monitoring and evaluation would be integrated into an existing function rather than conducted separately.

Another consideration in deciding who, where, and how data will be collected is the level of knowledge required to collect the data. Some indicator data may be self-evident, while others may require some clinical knowledge to be collected reliably. For some indicators, medical record personnel, for example, could collect data, and for others some clinical assistance may be necessary.

Data collection can be retrospective or concurrent. Although some data must be collected retrospectively, concurrent data collection can be effective by using observation coupled with review of documents for timely communication of quality-related information and to minimize time involved in collecting the data. If sampling is appropriate for high-volume aspects of care and service, the sample size and sample-selection method should be established.

Those designing the data-collection methodology also will need to study the organization's computer capabilities. Computerized data collection, especially in larger hospitals, may speed the process. Computers can also be used to show when evaluation is triggered. And computers can display findings in various ways, including graphically and by units, shifts, departments, and types of patients.

The various structures, sizes, and computer capabilities of health care organizations make it unwise to require any one data-collection method. The organization should choose the method that works best for it.

Findings should be reported at specified times to the individual or group responsible for organizing the data and determining whether evaluation is triggered. This activity could be performed by those who generate this data, those who collect the data, a quality-improvement professional, or any other appropriate individual or group familiar with the way evaluation is triggered. Patterns/trends that trigger evaluation may be harder to apply than upper and lower limits or specific performance rates. The timing for reporting the results of data collection will depend on the aspect of care and service under consideration and organization resources, but typically will be monthly, bimonthly, quarterly, or semi-annually. Sentinel events are usually reported as they occur.

Other quality-related feedback. Those designing monitoring and evaluation should establish channels by which the leaders and others receive feedback that is not part of ongoing monitoring, but that is related to the quality of care and service. This feedback may come from surveys, comments, suggestions, and complaints of staff, patients, patients' families, and others who use the organization's services. This aspect of data collection (which is new in this description of monitoring and evaluation) recognizes that information from sources outside ongoing monitoring can and should be used to trigger further evaluation and efforts to improve care and service.

Step 7: Initiate Evaluation

A decision must be made whether the data, both from ongoing monitoring and other quality-related feedback, warrant further evaluation of the aspect of care and service.

Determining when to evaluate. At regular, specified times, the responsible individual(s) should assess the data to determine whether they indicate the need for further evaluation based on the established trends, patterns, limits, or levels. (According to the organization's plan for quality improvement, these individuals may also evaluate the care and service and take action.)

Setting priorities for evaluation. The individuals responsible should assess the findings from ongoing monitoring that trigger evaluation, as well as other feedback (for example, patient satisfaction surveys, staff comments) that suggests opportunities for improvement may be present. Then, taking into consideration the potential effect on patient care and service as well as organization resources, priorities for further evaluation are set.

Convening teams. Those individuals who can best evaluate all facets of the particular aspect(s) of care and service are then brought together. This team may be the same one that developed the indicators or another group with appropriate representation. When necessary, these teams should be composed of members from different departments and services, to assure that interdepartmental processes are considered.

Evaluating care and service. Evaluation, including peer review when appropriate, should be used to determine whether there is an opportunity to improve care or service. In general, staff evaluating care should be attentive to opportunities for improvement involving systems, knowledge, and behavior.

One difficulty in evaluating care and service is determining exactly how performance can be improved. It is important to make such decisions as objectively as possible. Many tools can facilitate objectivity and help teams understand the causes of observed performance. These include measures of processes and outcomes; cause-and-effect diagrams, pareto diagrams, flowcharts, run charts, control charts, histograms, and scatter diagrams; department standards, guidelines, protocols, and parameters of care or practice; the team members' expertise; professional society guidelines; and pertinent health care literature.

Teams should record in worksheets or minutes their assessment, conclusions, recommendations, and rationales.

As mentioned elsewhere in this book, monitoring and evaluation has often focused on finding isolated problems, including practitioners not performing up to standards. Certainly, one component of improving quality should be to help find and solve chronic problems, whether they involve systems, equipment, or personnel. But the greatest opportunities to improve quality do not lie in the errors people make; rather, they lie in improving the overall performance of the systems, equipment, and personnel—the continuous improvement of performance. Opportunities for such improvement are most often found in ongoing processes rather than in isolated individuals.

Step 8: Take Actions to Improve Care

If evaluation identifies an opportunity for improvement, actions should be recommended and taken.

Recommending action. The team evaluating the aspect of care or service should determine appropriate actions; depending on the aspect of care or service being evaluated, these teams may take actions themselves and forward the results to the leaders. Actions should be directed toward the root causes and should have an eye toward overall improvement in the quality of care and service.

Some possible actions include

- (for systems problems) changes in communication channels, changes in organizational structures and processes, adjustments in staffing, and changes in equipment or chart forms;
- (for knowledge problems) in-service education, continuing education, making data or scientific reports accessible, and circulating informational material; and
- (for individual skill problems) changes in assignments, informal or formal counseling, and disciplinary action.

Implementing actions. Under some circumstances, quality improvement teams and other staff may be empowered to select and implement actions. Under other circumstances, the leaders may be responsible for deciding which actions to implement and selecting who will implement them. The leaders may decide the teams themselves should take certain actions (for example, designing systems changes). Other actions may fall into the purview of department/service chairs or may require the formation of ad hoc groups.

Step 9: Assess the Effectiveness of Actions and Assure Improvement Is Maintained

Monitoring and evaluation does not end when actions are taken. Whether the actions actually improve care or service should be determined and the improvement should be maintained.

Subsequent findings. The findings from continued monitoring (or from special follow-up monitoring, for areas not subject to ongoing monitoring) will provide evidence to determine whether actions were effective. Data from one or two monitoring periods may be necessary to make the determination. If care and service do not improve within the expected time, responsible individuals could initiate further evaluation and determine further action. Responsible staff should be attentive to findings as they continue to be compiled; ongoing and follow-up monitoring should ultimately show that meaningful improvement is maintained.

Continue monitoring. Ongoing monitoring should continue for the selected important aspects of care and service. When feedback from outside the ongoing monitoring process triggers evaluation, the leaders should choose the appropriate follow-up monitoring. They may decide that, for example, subsequent patient-satisfaction questionnaires will provide sufficient information. They may also decide that ongoing monitoring needs to be initiated; then, a team would identify indicators, triggers, and data sources for the aspect of care, which would be added to the ongoing monitoring activities. The important aspects of care that have been chosen for ongoing monitoring should be regularly reviewed to determine whether the priorities for monitoring should be changed or whether indicators should be revised.

Step 10: Communicate Results to Relevant Individuals and Groups

To "close the loop" of monitoring and evaluation, the conclusions, recommendations, actions, and follow-up must be reported to the appropriate individuals and groups.

The involved team, as well as the organization leaders, should disseminate necessary information throughout the organization. In addition, the leaders and others will receive formal and informal comments, reactions, and information from involved individuals and groups on the effectiveness of monitoring and evaluation. These should also be made known to affected individuals and groups.

MODIFICATIONS TO THE PROCESS

The monitoring and evaluation process described builds on that required by Joint Commission standards through 1991. The modifications involve, primarily,

- emphasizing the leadership role in improving quality;
- expanding the scope of assessment and improvement activities beyond the strictly clinical to the interrelated governance, managerial, support, and clinical processes that affect patient outcomes;
- using other sources of feedback (in addition to ongoing monitoring) to trigger evaluation and improvement of care and service;
- organizing the assessment and improvement activities around the flow of patient care and service, with special attention to how the "customer and supplier" relationships between departments (as well as within departments) can be improved, rather than compartmental-

izing activities within departments and services;

- focusing first on the processes of care and service rather than solely on the performance of individuals;
- emphasizing continuous improvement rather than only solving identified problems; and
- maintaining improvement over time.

The monitoring and evaluation process continues to provide for ongoing assessment and improvement of care and service; the modifications allow the process to be more comprehensive, more clearly defined, and more effective in improving care and service for the patients of a health care organization.

OTHER METHODS FOR ASSESSMENT AND IMPROVEMENT

In the next sections are several other assessment and improvement processes, culled from various sources. Readers are encouraged to go to the sources for more in-depth informatiion on these processes. Each of these can be successfully adapted for use in a health care organization within a program of continuous quality improvement. As of 1992, Joint Commission standards will not describe the ten-step monitoring and evaluation process explicitly, although many of its ten steps will remain in the standards. (See Appendix A for the 1992 "Quality Assessment and Improvement" standards.) In the 1994 standards, the methods for monitoring, assessing, and improving care will be even less prescriptive. As organizations make the transition to quality improvement, they may want to modify the ten-step monitoring and evaluation process or adopt another process that fits their system. It is likely that an effective process for monitoring, assessing, and improving care and service will fulfill the Joint Commission's 1992 standards, because most such processes will involve the steps listed in the standards (for example, selecting areas to monitor, collecting data, evaluating care and service), even if the sequence of the steps is not that of the ten-step monitoring and evaluation process.

Plan, Do, Check, Act[4]

The planning and improvement process that has perhaps the widest currency is the Shewart Cycle (named for Walter A. Shewart). It was introduced in Japan by W. Edwards Deming and so is often called the Deming Cycle. Currently, it is usually referred to as the PDCA cycle; those initials stand for the four components of the cycle: plan, do, check, act.

THE PLAN-DO-CHECK-ACT CYCLE FOR INDENTIFYING AND SOLVING PROBLEMS

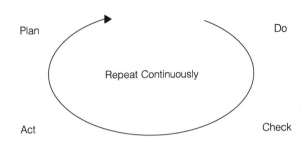

1. Plan change by studying a process, deciding what could improve it, and identifying data to help

2. Do test the proposed change by data stimulatiion or small-scale trial.

3. Check the effects by studying the results; modify the planned change if necessary.

4. Act to improve the process by implementing change.

Source: Walton M: The Deming Management Method, 1986.

Figure 14

This cycle by which organizations continuously improve processes was introduced in Japan by W. Edwards Deming.

Like monitoring and evaluation, PDCA is an ongoing process designed to direct study, action, reassessment, and further action.

The *plan* step involves studying a process by collecting the necessary data and evaluating the results. The evaluation should result in a plan for improvement. In the *do* step, the plan is carried out on a small scale or by simulation. Staff next observe or *check* the results of the change. Based on the results, the next step is to *act*—to implement change to improve the process. These steps are repeated, to increase knowledge and improvement.

The PDCA cycle corresponds primarily to steps 7 through 10 in the 10-step process described previously in this chapter. Steps 2 through 6 of the 10-step process are a method for determining the object of the PDCA cycle.

Figure 14 illustrates the PDCA cycle.

FOCUS-PDCA

The Hospital Corporation of America preceded the PDCA cycle with its FOCUS strategy. FOCUS is an acronym for Find, Organize, Clarify, Understand, and Select. *Find* means to chose a process that needs to be improved. *Organize* involves putting together a team of people knowledgeable in the process. *Clarify* means to assemble and review the current knowledge of the process. To *understand* requires measuring the process and learning the causes of variation. The team then must *select* the major cause of variation, thus focusing attention on a specific problem. The PDCA cycle then allows the team to formulate and implement actions to improve the process and to assess the effectiveness of the actions.

Steps 2 through 6 of the 10-step process help identify the subject to be focused on—the "F" portion of the process. The "OCUS" portion of FOCUS-PCDA corresponds to step 7 in the 10-step model and leads to an effective PDCA cycle (steps 7 to 10 in the 10-step process) by providing for the involvement of the right people, the understanding of the process, and the use of good measures to make appropriate plans for process improvement.

The Hospital Corporation of America's depiction of this process is shown in Figure 15.

Juran's "Journey"[5]

Joseph Juran groups the activities of a quality-improvement team into two categories: the diagnostic journey and the remedial journey.

The diagnostic journey. This portion of the problem-solving process moves from the evidence of the problem toward identifying its cause. At least these three activities are involved:

1. *Understanding the symptom.* This step requires not only noting the words and findings that indicate a problem exists, but investigating to learn, as specifically as possible, the *symptoms.*
2. *Theorizing as to causes.* Juran suggests that those affected by the problem brainstorm and organize the various theories that result.
3. *Testing the theories.* This testing may require small-scale or large-scale data collection and analysis and should result in identifying the symptoms' cause or causes.

The remedial journey. This journey moves from the causes to their remedy. The activities involved include these three:

1. *Stimulating the establishment of a remedy.* Although the project team itself may not establish the remedy, Juran suggests that the team "follow up and stimulate until the remedy has been established."
2. *Testing the remedy under operating conditions.* This activity involves implementing and observing the remedy under day-to-day conditions. Juran encourages the project team to make sure "the cure is not worse than the disease."
3. *Establishing controls to hold the gains.* Juran reminds that "[some] changes are reversible." Whatever procedures are necessary to make sure improvement is maintained should be implemented.

While steps 2 through 6 in the 10-step process help identify the subject for the diagnostic journey, the diagnostic and remedial journeys are similar to steps 7 through 10 of the 10-step process.

A Five-Stage Plan for Process Improvement[6]

Joiner and Associates, a quality consultant in Madison, Wisconsin, promulgates a five-stage plan for process improvement in its book The Team Handbook. The stages are as follows:

- Stage 1: *Understand the process.* In this stage, a team studies the process in question, describing it, noting customer needs, and coming up with a standard.
- Stage 2: *Eliminate errors.* This stage requires making changes necessary to remove continuing errors that have been noted in the process.
- Stage 3: *Remove slack.* To carry out this stage, the team looks for ways to remove unnecessary steps or otherwise streamline the process.
- Stage 4: *Reduce variation.* Next, it is necessary to identify and reduce common causes and special causes. (Common and special causes are discussed in Chapter Four under the section on control charts.) This action should bring the process under statistical control.
- Stage 5: *Plan for continuous improvement.* In this stage, having eliminated the prominent problems, the team formulates a process to continuously study and improve the process, using the PDCA cycle.

This process, like the others, makes use of statistical quality control techniques and the theories of Deming, Juran, et al.

FADE

The FADE process has been described by Organizational Dynamics, Inc., a consulting firm in Boston that specializes

THE FOCUS PROCESS FOR QUALITY IMPROVEMENT

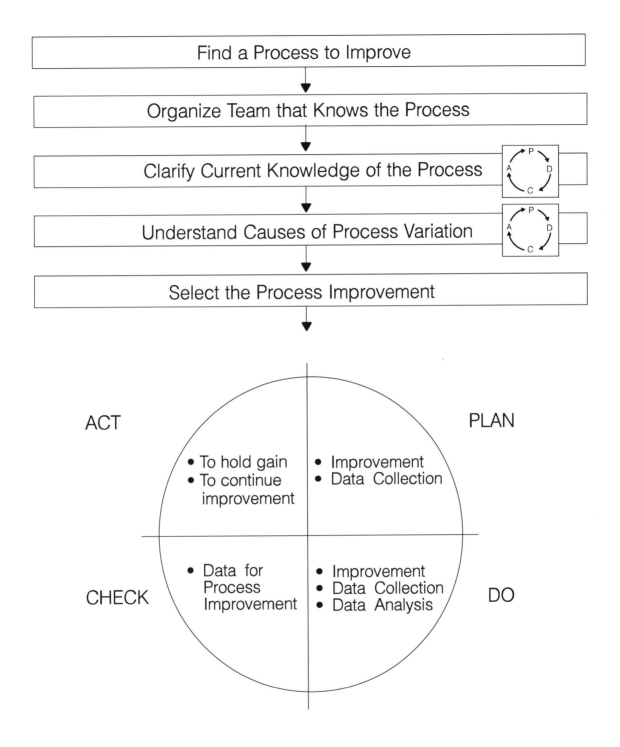

Figure 15
This illustration shows the FOCUS process—by which organizations select a process to improve—leading into Deming's
Plan-Do-Check-Act Cycle. **Source:** The Hospital Corporation of America. Used with permission.

in quality improvement. The steps of this process, shown in Figure 16, are Focus, Analyze, Develop, and Execute. To *focus*, a team narrows a list of problems to one, verifies the problem, and articulates it in a written statement. The next step, *analyze*, includes collecting data and determining "influential factors." *Develop* means developing a plan to solve the problem. Finally, to *execute*, the team gains an organizational commitment, puts the plan into action, and monitors its effect.

Evangelical Health Systems

In its CQI [continuous quality improvement] Monitoring System, Evangelical Health Systems has linked the Joint Commission's ten-step monitoring and evaluation process with terms more common to quality improvement literature and practices. They divide monitoring and evaluation into five phases: planning, measurement, feedback and evaluation, action, and reporting.

Planning includes the first five steps of the ten-step process, which help identify who, what, and how—who will oversee and perform the monitoring, what will be monitored, and how it will be monitored. *Measurement* entails step 6—collecting and organizing data to note significant variations. *Feedback and evaluation* include steps 7 and 9. Step 7 is the evaluation of care when warranted by the data, and step 9 asks that the effects of corrective action be monitored. The *action* phase comprises step 8 of the monitoring and evaluation process—taking action based on the evaluation. And *reporting* includes step 10—communicating the results of monitoring and evaluation to appropriate individuals and groups.

Figure 17 shows how this process is expressed graphically.

EXAMPLE[7]

It would be helpful to walk through one example of how these quality improvement processes work. For simplicity's sake, the process used will be divided into four parts: measurement, evaluation, action, and follow-up.

Measurement

One special concern for the alcohol and other drug dependence unit of this hypothetical hospital was the ability of multiple-relapse patients to identify and understand the effects of their relapse triggers. This information is recorded in the patient record during routine reassessments and at discharge. It is also plotted during weekly case review on a control chart showing percent of patients able to identify and understand relapse triggers. The upper specification limit for this indicator was set at 90% and the lower limit at 70%

The clinical coordinator and the medical director, both of whom reviewed findings monthly, noted that the performance had moved steadily toward the lower limit and decided to take action.

Evaluation

Because of the importance of this aspect of treatment, a team was called together consisting of a registered nurse, two alcohol and drug clinicians, an addiction counselor, and a physician consultant. Using a cause-and-effect diagram to guide their discussion, the team noted the surprisingly varied and numerous actions that led to a patient identifying his or her relapse triggers. The staff also collected data to ascertain why the performance rate may be slipping now. They used a scatter diagram to analyze the relationship between knowledge of relapse triggers and a number of other variables, including staffing levels, turnover rate, and the unit's patient population.

As a result of this study, the team tentatively identified two causes for the difficulty—a "special cause" and a "common cause." The decrease in ability to identify relapse triggers matched a recent rise in patient population as a result of a new marketing campaign. This was believed to be the special cause resulting in the recent drop below the control limit. The common cause had to do with documentation. An especially important and problematic "hand off" shown in the cause-and-effect diagram was the documentation in the medical history of the patient's previous attempts to maintain abstinence, response to previous treatment, and history of relapses. It was widely assumed that the admitting physicians were aware of the importance of this information, but the way it was documented often made it difficult to ascertain: it was often integrated into the narrative history and was often not highlighted in the summary or elsewhere in the assessment. Further investigation showed that relapse triggers identified in the medical history often were not addressed in the initial treatment plan; therefore, relapse triggers were inadequately addressed in treatment. The quality of the documentation was otherwise high, but the consulting physician, nurse, clinicians, and counselors all noted that the form did not suggest the need to highlight this information, nor did it provide a space for such highlighting.

THE FADE PROCESS FOR QUALITY IMPROVEMENT

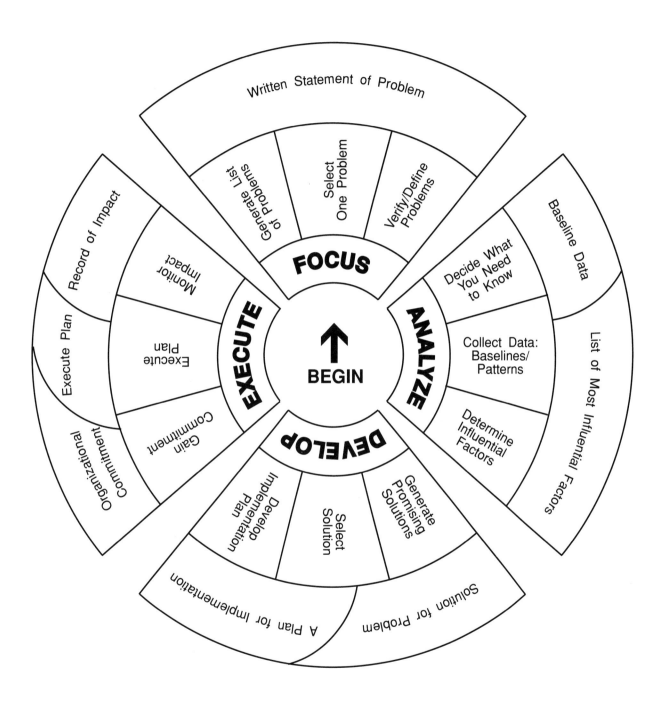

Figure 16
The FADE process encourages organizations to FOCUS on a problem, ANALYZE it,
DEVELOP a plan for improvement, and EXECUTE the plan.
Source: Organizational Dynamics, Inc Used with permission.

Action

The team quickly drafted a revised assessment form to help physicians highlight this important information both in the medical history and in the assessment summary. The form was approved by the alcohol and drug unit and by the medical record department; a small number were printed and they were tested for two months.

Follow-up

After two months, data showed that performance for this indicator was consistently within the specification limits. Review of patient records showed that the treatment plans of the patients admitted within that month all addressed the specified relapse triggers; in addition, 85% of those patients who had progressed far enough in treatment to do so understood their relapse triggers. The team discussed these findings and concluded that these positive results warranted

implementation of the new assessment form. New forms were printed, and education was provided to all physicians and relevant staff on their use. Continued monitoring would be conducted to see whether the variation in performance continued to be reduced and the overall rate continued to be within specification limits.

SUMMARY

Looking closely at the various improvement processes in this chapter shows they have much in common. They all involve some way of selecting a process or aspect of care to assess, measuring it, evaluating it, taking action to improve it, and assessing the results. Such a process, no matter how many steps or what its acronym, must be grounded in statistical methods, collecting data reliably and displaying them in such a way as to show the need for improvement.

TEN-STEP MONITORING AND EVALUATION PROCESS FOR QUALITY IMPROVEMENT

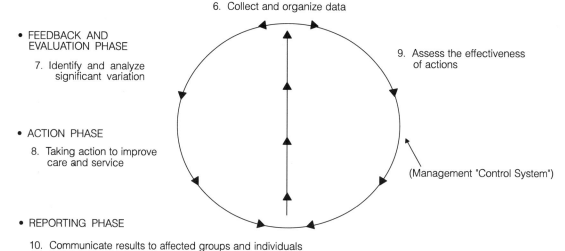

- PLANNING PHASE

    1. Assign responsibility
    2. Delineate scope of care and service
    3. Identify important aspects of care and service
    4. Identify indicators
    5. Establish evaluation triggers

- MEASUREMENT PHASE

    6. Collect and organize data

- FEEDBACK AND EVALUATION PHASE

    7. Identify and analyze significant variation

    9. Assess the effectiveness of actions

- ACTION PHASE

    8. Taking action to improve care and service

    (Management "Control System")

- REPORTING PHASE

    10. Communicate results to affected groups and individuals

Figure 17
This figure organizes the ten-step monitoring and evaluation process into five phases—planning, measurement, feedback and evaluation, action, and reporting. **Source:** Adapted from Evangelical Health Systems. Used with permission.

:hnology, 1986.

:rship for Quality. New York: The

Handbook. Madison, Wisconsin:
1989.

provement from: Weedman RD:
ng and evaluation in alcoholism
ence services, in Monitoring and
n and Other Drug Dependence
Commission on Accreditation of
ns, 1987.

Chapter Six

IN SUMMARY

As a way of revisiting the principles of quality improvement in health care, offering tips on implementing quality improvement, and casting a glance at its possibilities, this chapter takes another look at the National Demonstration Project on Quality Improvement in Health Care.[1] This project, as mentioned previously, involved 21 health care organizations in specific projects to test the applicability of quality improvement methods to health care. Of the 21 projects, 15 were considered successful. From the experiences, ten "key lessons" are reported in the book Curing Health Care. The lessons of those who have grappled with quality improvement offer valuable insight into the benefits and challenges of this technique of improving health care quality.

Lesson 1: *Quality improvement tools can work in health care.* The high success rate alone offers persuasive evidence that quality improvement works in health care. The experience of individual teams supports the conclusion. Most found that quality-control tools allowed new insights into the processes involved. One team wrote,

The theories and tools of statistically based total quality control and the framework for using the tools, including involvement of all levels of an organization and cutting across functional departmental lines, were readily accepted and successfully introduced....the emphasis on statistical education may be more easily spread in health care organizations than in other industries due to the scientific and technical education that the majority of health care workers have had in their professional training.

Lesson 2: *Cross-functional teams are valuable in improving health care processes.* The advice of quality experts to concentrate on communication across departmental lines, on internal customer-supplier relationships, proved sound for these health care organizations. Study of the complex steps that made up the processes under consideration required communication between the diverse individuals involved in those processes. In turn, respect for and understanding of the interdependencies in the organizations arose. Improved quality was the result.

Lesson 3: *Data useful for quality improvement abound in health care*. The project teams found, generally, that the data they needed were already available. Data recording is an ingrained part of health care organizations; the teams found these available data useful in their quality improvement projects. Often, simple changes in the way available data were organized helped identify opportunities for improvement.

Lesson 4: *Quality improvement methods are fun to use.* Participants reported a sense of purpose and accomplishment in their use of quality improvement methods to improve health care. Deming equates this state of mind with the culture needed to champion quality.

Lesson 5: *Costs of poor quality are high, and savings are within reach*. Many of the projects found poor quality resulted in significant costs. For example, "[a]t the Massachusetts Respiratory Hospital, costs of agency nurses to fill in for missing nursing staff were well over $20,000 per month." At the end of the project, "agency nursing bills fell by 42 percent, and net nursing salary costs fell by $7,500 per week." The evidence from the National Demonstration Project is not conclusive, but shows the high cost of poor quality and suggests the possibility of saving money through use of quality improvement techniques.

Lesson 6: *Involving doctors is difficult*. Busy schedules and skepticism can be barriers to physician involvement in quality improvement. Physicians may be especially reluctant when not full-time employees of the hospital. Physicians need to understand the direct benefits quality improvement can have for them, and they need to know that quality improvement is a new approach to quality that has left behind the negative baggage of quality assurance.

Lesson 7: *Training needs arise early*. Those project participants who have subsequently chosen to implement quality improvement in their organizations have found training an immediate need. To acquire the training, they have faced the difficult task of choosing from among the various quality experts as consultants, or setting up their own internal educational resources. Some cities and regions have established networks with non-health care companies to learn about quality improvement techniques.

Lesson 8: *Nonclinical processes draw early attention*. Nonclinical areas, such as staffing, tend to be safe places to begin quality improvement. Although such areas can affect patient outcomes, it is important to recognize that these systems and the processes of clinical care work together. Reluctance to address clinical care directly can result in loss of vital inputs to quality improvement; after all, nonclinical and clinical processes intertwine in a health care organization and must be addressed as such if quality improvement is to have an effect.

Lesson 9: *Health care organizations may need a broader definition of quality*. Quality improvement in industry focuses on quality as fulfilling customer needs. Project participants often had difficulty integrating this impression of quality with the impression of quality as pertaining "almost exclusively to hands-on medical care." One organization suggests, "The biggest obstacle to systems-wide implementation of these techniques in health care may be ambiguity, especially in academic health care facilities, about the collective definition of 'quality' itself..."

Lesson 10: *In health care, as in industry, the fate of quality improvement is first of all in the hands of leaders*. Of the health care organizations involved in the National Demonstration Project, those with the strongest top management support saw the greatest success. "In fact, *every* project report commented on the importance of visible senior management support in the work of quality improvement." Quality improvement requires resources, planning, and constancy of mission; these must start with upper management.

These ten lessons reenforce some of the important principles of quality assurance: use of quality-control tools, removal of communication barriers, focus on processes, importance of training, and importance of leadership commitment. They also point to some looming challenges: involving physicians and leaders, defining quality, addressing clinical issues. But perhaps most important, these lessons offer an optimistic view for the future: quality improvement engenders a sense of purpose in participants and actually can improve the quality of care and services in health care.

REFERENCE

1. Information and quotations in this chapter are drawn from: Berwick DM et al: Curing Health Care: New Strategies for Quality Improvement, A report on the National Demonstration Project on Quality Improvement in Health Care. San Francisco: Jossey-Bass Publishers, 1990.

Appendix A

'QUALITY ASSESSMENT AND IMPROVEMENT' CHAPTER FROM THE 1992 ACCREDITATION MANUAL FOR HOSPITALS

PREAMBLE

This chapter—formerly called "Quality Assurance"—describes the activities of the hospital that are designed to assess and improve the quality of patient care. The chapter includes revisions and additions to the 1991 standards, which are intended to assist hospitals in performing these activities more effectively. The standards revisions are focused on the following two areas:

- placing greater emphasis on the role of the hospital's leaders—governance, managerial, medical, nursing, and other clinical leaders—in assessing and improving patient care; and
- shifting the emphases and further clarifying certain steps in the monitoring and evaluation process.

In addition, in an effort to simplify this Manual, some standards related to quality assessment and improvement that were repeated in numerous other chapters of this Manual have been consolidated into this chapter (and deleted from the others).

The revised standards are based on the following principles:

- A hospital can improve patient care quality—that is, increase the probability of desired patient outcomes, including patient satisfaction—by assessing and improving those governance, managerial, clinical, and support processes that most affect patient outcomes.
- Some of these processes are carried out by medical, nursing, and other clinicians, some by governing body members, some by managers, and some by support personnel; some are carried out jointly by more than one of these groups.
- Whether carried out by one or more groups, the processes must be coordinated and integrated; this coordination and integration requires the attention of the managerial and clinical leaders of the hospital.
- Most governance, managerial, medical, nursing, other clinical, and support staff are both motivated and competent to carry out the processes well. Therefore, the opportunities to improve the processes—and, thus, improve patient outcomes—are much more frequent than are mistakes and errors. Consequently, without shirking its responsibility to address serious problems involving deficits in knowledge or skill, the hospital's principal goal should be to help everyone improve the processes in which he/she is involved.

These principles underlie the continuous assessment and improvement of quality. For hospitals, the natural next step in the steady progression of approaches from implicit peer review, to medical audits, to systematic quality assurance (QA), is to continuous improvement of quality.

Beginning with this 1992 Manual and progressing over the next few years, the Joint Commission is incrementally revising the standards on quality assessment and improvement to help hospitals use their current commitment, resources, and approaches to improving patient care quality more effectively and efficiently. The revisions in this Manual are designed to emphasize the role of hospital leaders in these quality improvement activities, to encourage hospitals to evaluate their current activities in light of the above principles, and to assist those hospitals that are already moving toward the continuous improvement of quality. In subsequent editions of this Manual, the standards revisions will begin to establish expectations for all hospitals to continuously improve quality.

New to the chapter this year is a series of standards (QA.1 through QA.1.6) that addresses the important role that the hospital's leaders play collectively and individually in assessing and improving patient care quality. These standards emphasize the governance, managerial, medical, nursing, and other clinical leaders' responsibilities to set expectations for quality assessment and improvement, to provide the resources and training needed for these activities, to foster communication and coordination, and to personally participate in improvement activities.

The revisions in the monitoring and evaluation standards are intended to shift some emphases of the previous standards in order to help hospitals overcome common weaknesses in current QA practice that can inhibit the development of an approach to continuously assessing and improving quality. These common weaknesses in current practice include

- a frequent focus on only the clinical aspects of care (for example, what the doctor and nurse do with the patient), rather than on the full series of interrelated governance, managerial, support, and clinical processes that affect patient outcomes;

- a frequent compartmentalization of QA activities in accordance with hospital structure (for example, by department, by discipline) rather than organizing quality improvement activities around the flow of patient care, in which the interrelated processes are often cross-disciplinary and cross-departmental;

- a frequent focus on only the performance of individuals, especially on problem performance, rather than on how well the processes in which they participate are performed, how well the processes are coordinated and integrated (for example, the "handoffs"), and how the processes can be improved;

- frequently initiating action only when a problem is identified, rather than also trying to find better ways to carry out processes; and

- separating the appropriateness ("Was the right thing done?") and effectiveness ("Was it done right?") of care from the efficiency of care, rather than integrating efforts to improve patient outcomes with those to improve efficiency (that is, improving value).

In addition, because of its frequent focus on only individual performance, especially problem performance, for many health care professionals current QA practice often has a negative persona that can interfere with their instinct to pursue lifelong self-assessment and constant professional growth.

The changes in the monitoring and evaluation standards are designed to shift the emphases of quality assessment and improvement activities away from an approach that is frequently department- and discipline-specific, direct care focused, and individual- and problem-oriented, to an approach that reflects the principles described above. This approach is expected to better harness the professional instinct for continuous improvement.

Please note that the phrase "monitoring and evaluation of the quality and appropriateness of care has been modified by deleting "and appropriateness," since contemporary definitions of "quality" include "appropriateness" among the characteristics of quality (for example, effectiveness, appropriateness, accessibility, continuity, efficiency).

Note: In QA.1, only QA.1.1 will be surveyed for accreditation in 1992.

QA.1 The organization's leaders* set expectations, develop plans, and implement procedures to assess and improve the quality of the organization's governance, management, clinical, and support processes.

QA.1.1 The leaders undertake education concerning the approach and methods of continuous quality improvement.

QA.1.2 The leaders set priorities for organizationwide quality improvement activities that are designed to improve patient outcomes.

QA.1.3 The leaders allocate adequate resources for assessment and improvement of the organization's governance, managerial, clinical, and support processes, through

> **QA.1.3.1** the assignment of personnel, as needed, to participate in quality improvement activities;

> **QA.1.3.2** the provision of adequate time for personnel to participate in quality improvement activities; and

> **QA.1.3.3** information systems and appropriate data management processes to facilitate the collection, management, and analysis of data needed for quality improvement.

QA.1.4 The leaders assure that organization staff are trained in assessing and improving the processes that contribute to improved patient outcomes.

QA.1.5 The leaders individually and jointly develop and participate in mechanisms to foster communication among individuals and among components of the organization, and to coordinate internal activities.

QA.1.6 The leaders analyze and evaluate the effectiveness of their contributions to improving quality.

*The leaders responsible for performing the identified functions include at least the leaders of the governing body; the chief executive officer and other senior managers; the elected and appointed leaders of the medical staff and the clinical departments, and other medical staff members in hospital administrative positions; and the nursing executive and other senior nursing leaders.

QA.2 The organization has a written plan for assessing and improving quality that describes the objectives, organization, scope, and mechanisms for overseeing the effectiveness of monitoring, evaluation, and improvement activities. The plan includes at least the activities listed in QA.2.1 through QA.2.4.2 and described in other chapters of this Manual.

QA.2.1 The following medical staff quality assessment and improvement activities are performed:

QA.2.1.1 the assessment and improvement of the quality of patient care and the clinical performance of individuals with clinical privileges through

QA.2.1.1.1 participation by members of each department/service in intra- and/or interdepartmental/service monitoring and evaluation of care; periodic review of the care; and communication of findings, conclusions, recommendations, and actions to members of the department/service;

QA.2.1.1.2 evaluation and improvement in the use of surgical and other invasive procedures;

QA.2.1.1.3 evaluation and improvement in the use of medications;

QA.2.1.1.4 the medical record review function;

QA.2.1.1.5 evaluation and improvement in the use of blood and blood components; and

QA.2.1.1.6 the pharmacy and therapeutics function.

QA.2.2 The quality of patient care, including that provided to specific age groups, in all patient care services is monitored and evaluated.

QA.2.2.1 The departments/services in which care is monitored and evaluated include at least those addressed in other chapters in this Manual, when provided.

QA.2.2.2 The director of each department/service is responsible for including the department's/service's activities in the monitoring and evaluation process.

QA.2.2.2.1 The department/service participates in

QA.2.2.2.1.1 the identification of important aspects of care relevant to the department/service;

QA.2.2.2.1.2 the identification of indicators used to

monitor the quality of the important aspects of care; and

QA.2.2.2.1.3 the evaluation of the quality of care.

QA.2.2.3 When the hospital provides a patient care service for which there is no designated department/service, the organization's leaders assign responsibility for implementing a monitoring and evaluation process.

QA.2.2.3.1 When the hospital, in its care of patients, requires the services of another, off-site health care organization, the monitoring and evaluation process examines the appropriateness of the hospital's use of the services and the degree to which the services aid in its care of patients.

QA.2.3 The following hospitalwide quality assessment and improvement activities are performed:

QA.2.3.1 infection control (see IC.1 and IC.2);

QA.2.3.2 utilization review (see UR.1); and

QA.2.3.3 review of accidents, injuries, patient safety, and safety hazards (see PL.1, PL.1.3.1.2, PL.1.3.1.3, PL.1.3.1.4, and PL.1.4.3).

QA.2.4 Relevant results from the quality assessment activities listed in QA.2.1 through QA.2.3.3

QA.2.4.1 are used primarily to study and improve processes that affect patient care outcomes; and

QA.2.4.2 when relevant to the performance of an individual, are used as a component of the evaluation of individual capabilities (see MS.2.5.5, MS.2.5.5.3, NC.2.1.1, and GB.1.14).

QA.3 There is a planned, systematic, and ongoing process for monitoring, evaluating, and improving the quality of care and of key governance, managerial, and support activities that has the characteristics described in QA.3.1 through QA.3.1.7.2.

QA.3.1 Those aspects of care that are most important to the health and safety of the patients served are identified.

QA.3.1.1 These important aspects of care are those that

QA.3.1.1.1 occur frequently or affect large numbers of patients;

QA.3.1.1.2 place patients at risk of serious consequences or of deprivation of substantial benefit when

QA.3.1.1.2.1 the care is not provided correctly; or

QA.3.1.1.2.2 the care is not provided when indicated; or

QA.3.1.1.2.3 the care is provided when not indicated; and/or

QA.3.1.1.3 tend to produce problems for patients or staff.

QA.3.1.2 Indicators are identified to monitor the quality of important aspects of care.

QA.3.1.2.1 The indicators are related to the quality of care and may include clinical criteria (sometimes called "clinical standards," "practice guidelines," or "practice parameters.")

QA.3.1.2.1.1 These indicators are

QA.3.1.2.1.1.1 objective;

QA.3.1.2.1.1.2 measurable; and

QA.3.1.2.1.1.3 based on current knowledge and clinical experience.

QA.3.1.3 Data are collected for each indicator.

QA.3.1.3.1 The frequency of data collection for each indicator and the sampling of events or activities are related to

QA.3.1.3.1.1 the frequency of the event or activity monitored;

QA.3.1.3.1.2 the significance of the event or activity monitored; and

QA.3.1.3.1.3 the extent to which the important aspect of care monitored by the indicator has been demonstrated to be problem-free.

QA.3.1.4 The data collected for each indicator are organized so that situations in which an evaluation of the quality of care is indicated are readily identified.

QA.3.1.4.1 Such evaluations are prompted at a minimum by

QA.3.1.4.1.1 important single clinical events; or

QA.3.1.4.1.2 levels or patterns/trends in care or outcomes that are at significant variance with predetermined levels and/or patterns/trends in care or outcomes.

QA.3.1.4.2 Such evaluations may also be initiated by comparison of the hospital's performance with that of other organizations ("benchmarking").

QA.3.1.4.3 Such evaluations may also be initiated when there is a desire to improve overall performance.

QA.3.1.5 When initiated, the evaluation of an important aspect of care

QA.3.1.5.1 includes a more detailed analysis of patterns/trends in the data collected on the indicators;

QA.3.1.5.2 is designed to identify opportunities to improve, or problems in, the quality of care; and

QA.3.1.5.3 includes review by peers when analysis of the care provided by an individual practitioner is undertaken.

QA.3.1.6 When an important opportunity to improve, or a problem in, the quality of care is identified,

QA.3.1.6.1 action is taken to improve the care or to correct the problem; and

QA.3.1.6.2 the effectiveness of the action taken is assessed through continued monitoring of the care.

QA.3.1.7 The findings, conclusions, recommendations, actions taken, and results of the actions taken are

QA.3.1.7.1 documented; and

QA.3.1.7.2 reported through established channels.

QA.4 The administration and coordination of the hospital's approach to assessing and improving quality are designed to assure that the activities described in QA.4.1 through QA.4.4 are undertaken.

QA.4.1 Each of the quality and assessment and improvement activities outlined in QA.2 and QA.3 is performed appropriately and effectively.

QA.4.2 Necessary information is communicated among departments/services and/or professional disciplines when opportunities to improve patient care or problems involve more than one department/service and/or professional discipline.

QA.4.2.1 Information from departments/services and the

findings of discrete quality assessment and improvement activities are used to detect trends, patterns, opportunities to improve, or potential problems that affect more than one department/service and/or professional discipline.

QA.4.2.2 There are operational linkages between the risk management functions related to the clinical aspects of patient care and safety and quality assessment and improvement function.

QA.4.2.3 Existing information from risk management activities that may be useful in identifying opportunities to improve the quality of patient care and/or resolve clinical problems is accessible to the quality assessment and improvement function.

QA.4.3 The status of identified opportunities or problems is tracked to assure improvement or resolution.

QA.4.4 The objectives, scope, organization, and effectiveness of the activities to assess and improve quality are evaluated at least annually and revised as necessary.

Appendix B

MEDICAL STAFF STANDARDS
FOR REVIEW OF SURGICAL AND OTHER INVASIVE PROCEDURES, EFFECTIVE MEDICATION USE, AND BLOOD AND BLOOD COMPONENTS FROM THE 1992 ACCREDITATION MANUAL FOR HOSPITALS

SURGICAL AND OTHER INVASIVE PROCEDURES

MS.5.1.2 Review of Surgical and Other Invasive Procedures.

MS.5.1.2.1 Review of surgical and other invasive procedures is conducted monthly by those departments/services performing such procedures or by a medical staff committee(s).

MS.5.1.2.2 The purpose of such review is to continuously improve the selection (appropriateness) and performance (effectiveness) of surgical and other invasive procedures.

MS.5.1.2.3 Categories of procedures are reviewed through the use of screening criteria to identify single cases or patterns of cases that require more intensive evaluation; and/or through intensive evaluation of a single case or group of cases.

MS.5.1.2.3.1 In identifying categories of procedures for review, priority is given to those categories that are performed in high volume, and/or are of high risk to patients, and/or are suspected or known to be problem prone.

MS.5.1.2.3.2 Screening criteria are predetermined and may apply to either one specific category of procedure or to several categories of procedures.

MS.5.1.2.3.2.1 When the review of specimens removed during a surgical or other invasive procedure (described in PA.6.1.1 through PA.6.1.1.3) identifies a major discrepancy, or a pattern of discrepancies, between preoperative and postoperative (including pathologic) diagnoses, intensive evaluation is performed.

MS.5.1.2.3.3 When screening or intensively evaluating any category of procedure, an adequate number of cases is included.

MS.5.1.2.3.4 The combined use of screening mechanisms and intensive evaluation encompasses most categories of surgical and other invasive procedures performed in the hospital.

MS.5.1.2.3.4.1 All categories of procedures that meet the criteria in MS.5.1.2.3.1 are encompassed by the review (except, for example, a high-volume procedure that is neither high risk nor problem prone).

MS.5.1.2.4 Relevant results from the review of surgical and other invasive procedures are used primarily to study and improve processes involved in the selection and performance of these procedures.

MS.5.1.2.5 When an individual has performance problems that he/she is unable or unwilling to improve, modifications are made in clinical privileges or job assignments as indicated or some other appropriate action(s) is taken.

MS.5.1.2.6 Written reports of conclusions, recommendations, actions taken, and the results of actions taken are maintained.

EFFECTIVE MEDICATION USE

MS.5.1.3 Drug Usage Evaluation.

MS.5.1.3.1 Drug usage evaluation is performed by the medical staff as a criteria-based, ongoing, planned and systematic process designed to continuously improve the appropriate and effective use of drugs.

MS.5.1.3.1.1 This process includes the routine collection and assessment of information in order to identify opportunities to improve the use of drugs and to resolve problems in their use.

MS.5.1.3.2 There is ongoing monitoring and evaluation of selected drugs that are chosen for one or more of the following reasons:

MS.5.1.3.2.1 The drug(s) is one of the most frequently prescribed drugs.

MS.5.1.3.2.2 The drug(s) is known or suspected to present a significant risk to patients.

MS.5.1.3.2.3 Use of the drug(s) is known or suspected to be problem-prone.

MS.5.1.3.2.4 The drug(s) is a critical component of the care provided for a specific diagnosis, condition, or procedure.

MS.5.1.3.3 The process for monitoring and evaluating the use of drugs

MS.5.1.3.3.1 is performed by the medical staff in cooperation with, as required, the pharmaceutical department/service, the nursing department/service, management and administrative staff, and other departments/services and individuals;

MS.5.1.3.3.2 is based on the use of objective criteria that reflect current knowledge, clinical experience, and relevant literature; and

MS.5.1.3.3.3 may include the use of screening mechanisms to identify, for more intensive evaluation, problems in or opportunities to improve the use of a specific drug or category of drugs.

MS.5.1.3.4 Relevant results from the drug usage evaluation are used primarily to study and improve processes that affect the appropriate and effective use of drugs.

MS.5.1.3.5 When an individual has performance problems that he/she is unable or unwilling to improve, modifications are made in clinical privileges or job assignments as indicated or some other appropriate action(s) is taken.

MS.5.1.3.6 Written reports of the findings, conclusions, recommendations, actions taken, and results of actions taken are maintained and reported at least quarterly through channels established by the medical staff.

BLOOD AND BLOOD COMPONENTS
MS.5.1.5 Blood Usage Review.

MS.5.1.5.1 The medical staff performs blood usage review at least quarterly to continuously improve the appropriateness and effectiveness with which blood and blood components are used.

MS.5.1.5.2 Blood usage review includes the following:

MS.5.1.5.2.1 the review of all categories of blood and blood components in the hospital;

MS.5.1.5.2.1.1 The use of each category of blood and blood components is reviewed through the use of screening criteria to identify single cases or patterns of cases that require more intensive evaluation; and/or through intensive evaluation of a single case or of a group of cases.

MS.5.1.5.2.1.1.1 Screening criteria are predetermined and may apply to either one specific category of blood or blood component or to several categories of blood or blood components.

MS.5.1.5.2.1.1.2 When screening or intensively evaluating any category of blood or blood component, an adequate number of cases is included.

MS.5.1.5.2.2 the intensive evaluation of all confirmed transfusion reactions;

MS.5.1.5.2.3 the development or approval of policies and procedures relating to the distribution, handling, use, and administration of blood and blood components;

MS.5.1.5.2.4 the review of the adequacy of transfusion services to meet the needs of patients; and

MS.5.1.5.2.5 the review of ordering practices for blood and blood components.

MS.5.1.5.3 Relevant results from the blood usage review are used primarily to study and improve processes that affect the appropriate and effective use of blood and blood components.

MS.5.1.5.4 When an individual has performance problems that he/she is unable or unwilling to improve, modifications are made in clinical privileges or job assignments as indicated or some other appropriate action(s) is taken.

MS.5.1.5.5 Written reports of conclusions, recommendations, actions taken, and the results of actions taken are maintained and reported.

Appendix C

CONCEPTS FOR QUALITY:
SOME IDEAS ON THE FUTURE DIRECTION OF JOINT COMMISSION QUALITY ASSESSMENT AND IMPROVEMENT STANDARDS

1994 will witness the continued transformation of Joint Commission quality assessment and improvement (QA) standards. This appendix presents some ideas on the direction of future QA standards, and describes the kinds of issues that will be addressed in the 1994 QA standards for the Accreditation Manual for Hospitals (AMH). We invite your thoughts and comments on the ideas and issues described in this appendix. Address them to the Director of the Department of Standards at the Joint Commission.

EXPECTATIONS AND UNDERLYING CONCEPTS

The 1994 QA standards for the AMH will more fully incorporate principles and techniques that foster continuous improvement in performance and quality, and will be constructed around several expectations. First, that a commitment to continuously improve the quality of patient care is woven throughout the organization, appearing in strategic planning, resource allocation, role expectations, reward structures, performance evaluations, and the organization's role in the community.

Second, that the organization has implemented an ongoing, comprehensive self-assessment mechanism that supports and promotes continuous improvement in the quality of patient care. This mechanism should be designed to elicit feedback on the quality of care from patients as well as practitioners, from payors as well as other organizational care providers, and from employees as well as the community.

And third, that, as part of the organization's self-assessment mechanism, a system of ongoing monitoring and evaluation of clinical and organizational performance has been implemented to provide information to support improvement in the effective and efficient performance of those processes that are important to the quality of patient care.

The 1994 QA standards will fall into the following five categories:
- leadership responsibility for improving quality;
- methods for improving performance and quality;
- education and training;
- communication and collaboration; and

- evaluation and effectiveness of activities to improve performance and quality.

The concepts upon which the standards for each of the five sections will be based are described in detail below.

LEADERSHIP RESPONSIBILITY FOR QUALITY IMPROVEMENT

An organization's leaders* are responsible for setting expectations, developing plans, and implementing procedures to assess and improve the quality of the organization's governance, management, clinical, and support processes.

Leadership fulfills these responsibilities by
- undertaking education concerning the approach and methods of continuous quality improvement;
- setting priorities for organizationwide quality improvement activities that are designed to improve patient outcomes;
- allocating adequate resources for assessment and improvement of the organization's governance, managerial, clinical, and support processes through
- the assignment of personnel, as needed, to participate in quality improvement activities,
- providing adequate time for personnel to participate in quality improvement activities, and
- creating information systems and appropriate data management processes to facilitate the collection, management, and analysis of data needed for quality improvement;
- assuring that organization staff are trained in assessing and improving the processes that contribute to improved patient outcomes;

The leaders responsible for performing the identified functions include at least the leaders of the governing body; the chief executive officer and other senior managers; the elected and appointed practitioner leaders of the medical staff and the clinical departments, and other medical staff members in hospital administrative positions; and the nursing executive(s) and other senior nursing leaders.

- developing and participating in, both individually and jointly, mechanisms to foster communication among individuals and among components of the organization and to coordinate internal activities; and
- analyzing and evaluating the effectiveness of their contributions to improve quality.

METHODS FOR IMPROVING PERFORMANCE AND QUALITY

Important functions (that is, those sets of processes that affect patient outcomes most significantly) throughout the organization are to be continuously assessed and improved. This is accomplished through

- ongoing monitoring of important functions;
- the use of other feedback, such as information from patient surveys;
- priority setting to target those functions to be assessed and improved; and
- assessing and improving the targeted functions.

ONGOING MONITORING OF IMPORTANT FUNCTIONS

Certain important functions should be monitored on an ongoing basis. The functions monitored should be those that

- affect large numbers of patients, and/or
- are significant for individual patients or patient groups, and
- are identified as important functions in the standards in the AMH.

Once the functions to be monitored are identified and prioritized, the organization selects indicators for the high-priority functions and collects data on them on an ongoing basis. These indicators should be either measures of patient outcomes that are believed to be correlated with a high-priority function, or measures of processes that are believed to be correlated with patient outcomes. Periodically, the organization should review this data to determine when a high-priority function is not consistent with expected patterns of processes or outcomes. This determination is used to set priorities for assessment and improvement activities.

OTHER FEEDBACK

In addition to ongoing monitoring, the organization seeks and uses feedback from patients, their families, practitioners, employees, purchasers, insurers, suppliers, and other health care organizations. Such feedback should be relevant to the quality of patient care and services provided. At least the following mechanisms are used to gather feedback:

- surveys of patients, their families, and other users of the organization's services; and
- ongoing review and follow-up of comments, complaints, and suggestions for improvement, as indicated. This feedback is used to set priorities for assessment and improvement activities.

PRIORITY SETTING FOR ASSESSMENT AND IMPROVEMENT

Functions to be assessed and improved are selected on the basis of the following considerations:

- a monitored important function that is not consistent with the expected patterns of processes or outcomes;
- a monitored important function that is consistent with the expected patterns of processes or outcomes, but whose performance could be improved;
- another function, not routinely monitored, that affects patient outcomes and that is not consistent with expected patterns of processes or outcomes; or
- another function, not routinely monitored, that affects patient outcomes and that is consistent with the expected patterns of processes or outcomes, but whose performance could be improved.

ASSESSMENT AND IMPROVEMENT

With the use of such tools as cause-and-effect diagrams, flowcharts, and measures of processes and of outcomes, the organization studies the processes that contribute to the function selected for assessment and improvement. A plan to improve the selected function is carried out by

- identifying the processes involved;
- determining the causes for variation in the processes and outcomes;
- identifying those process changes that could improve outcomes;
- planning process changes designed to improve outcomes,
- testing the process changes;
- measuring the process changes and their effect on outcomes;
- implementing the process changes if they improve performance; and
- taking action to assure that the observed improvement is maintained over time.

Sources of variation in specific processes and outcomes

are usually sought first in the design of the processes under evaluation, and then in the activities of individuals.

When variation in processes or outcomes is attributed to the activities of an individual, organizational processes that support the individual's activities are evaluated to identify whether improvements in these processes may have a positive effect on the individual's activities. When variation in the processes involve the activities of licensed independent practitioners, the medical staff is responsible for assuring that the processes are included in assessment and improvement activities.

When an individual's activities are deficient and the individual is unable (or unwilling) to improve his or her performance, changes are considered in the individual's role, responsibility, and/or status. These changes should be designed to improve processes and patient outcomes. The individual's explanation for his or her activities is considered in making decisions that would affect his or her role, responsibility, and/or status.

RESPONSIBILITY

The director or chief of each organizational component (for example, a department or service) is responsible for assuring that the processes in his or her component are included in the assessment and improvement activities.

All personnel in each organizational component are encouraged to make proposals at any time for improving processes within their own or others' components. Those involved in the component's activities participate in identifying the important processes to be assessed, identifying the indicators used to monitor the processes or their outcomes, and evaluating and improving the processes.

When, in its care of patients, the organization requires the services of another, off-site health care organization, the monitoring and evaluation process examines the appropriateness of the hospital's use of the services and the degree to which the services aid in its care of patients.

EDUCATION AND TRAINING

The organization provides for educational services, including information support, for its personnel. Educational services include the methods for improving performance and quality, continuing education, and human relations.

Methods to Improve Performance and Quality

Personnel are trained and educated in methods to assess and improve performance and quality and are provided with periodic training on topics related to such techniques. Training includes information on techniques for

- developing quality assessment measures,
- collecting data,
- performing appropriate statistical analyses,
- evaluating processes,
- developing useful reports,
- formulating conclusions to serve as the bases for recommendations and action, and
- developing proposals for actions designed to improve processes that contribute to patient outcomes.

Continuing Education

Personnel are provided access to continuing education and staff development programs, including opportunities to participate in relevant education programs outside the organization. Such education meets needs identified through the quality improvement activities.

Human Relations Training

Through such techniques as seminars, group discussions, and individual counseling, the organization works to sensitize all personnel, both clinical and non-clinical, to the fact that patients and staff may have differing cultural values, perceptions, and expectations about health, illness, health care, and quality of life.

Personnel are made aware of the emotional and social impact of illness and hospitalization on the patient and his or her family, and of the impact of their own personal and professional values and attitudes upon their interactions with patients. Moreover, personnel receive information concerning the cultural beliefs about illness and health care of those ethnic groups that are significantly represented among the patients served. And finally, all personnel who come into contact with patients are counseled to recognize, respect, and effectively deal with the values and cultural beliefs of their patients and themselves.

INFORMATION SUPPORT

The organization provides its personnel with access to current literature on clinical and management processes appropriate for use in the organization, medical ethics, and the impact of patient and clinical cultural systems upon health care management and the quality of care. In addition, the organization maintains or has access to a data base(s) showing its own performance and the performance of comparable organizations. Information contained in the data base(s) should be used for comparison and to provide benchmarks in improving processes and patient outcomes.

COMMUNICATION AND COLLABORATION

The organization develops mechanisms to facilitate communication among individuals and organizational components.

Minutes or reports of the meetings of such organization-wide committees and other bodies involved in planning, review, oversight, and decision making related to improving quality are distributed to relevant departments, services, and other organizational components in a timely manner. The heads of organizational components and the personnel under their supervision confer and collaborate with personnel from other organizational components on projects or tasks that will affect more than one component.

EVALUATION OF THE EFFECTIVENESS OF ACTIVITIES TO IMPROVE PERFORMANCE AND QUALITY

The organization evaluates the effectiveness of its activities to improve performance and quality and, at least annually, prepares a comprehensive report based on this evaluation.

Each organizational component submits an annual report indicating the status of all activities targeted for assessment and/or improvement during the previous year. These reports are used for planning future activities to improve performance and quality.